# OSCEsmart

## 50 Medical Student OSCEs in Anaesthetics & Critical Care

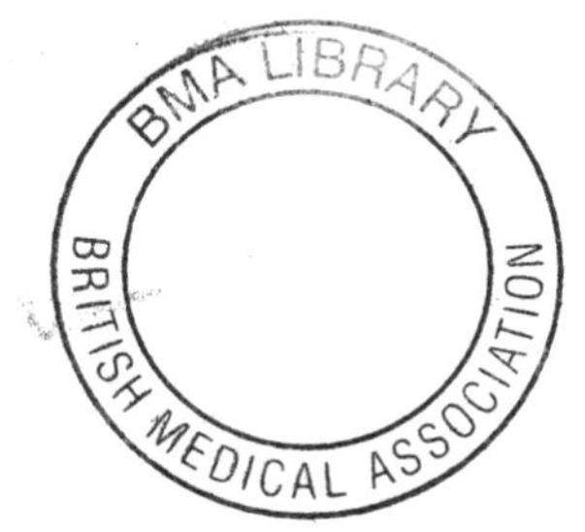


**Dr. Joe Lipton**

**Executive Consulting Editor:**
**Dr. Sam Thenabadu**

Ordering Information: Quantity sales. Special discounts are available on quantity purchases by corporations, associations, and others. For details, contact the publisher at the address above.

Orders by UK trade bookstores and wholesalers please visit www.scowenpublishing.com



Publisher's Cataloging-in-Publication data : OSCEsmart 50 medical student OSCEs in Anaesthetics & Critical Care



ISBN: 0-9908538-6-1

ISBN-13: 978-0-9908538-6-2

## DEDICATION

'For Sophie, Ted and Artie: the embarassing Liptoms'
**Joe**

'For Ammi, Molly, Reuben and Rafa - I.L.Y.T.T.M.'
**Sam**

# CONTENTS

# Message from the authors

Doctors of all seniorities can remember the stress of the OSCE but even more so the stress of trying to study and practice for the OSCEs. A multitude of generic undergraduate and postgraduate resources can be found on line but quality, quantity, and completeness of content can vary. The aim of the OSCESmart editorial team is to bring together specialty focused books that have identified 50 core stations encompassing the essential categories of history taking, examinations, emergency moulages, clinical skills and data interpretation with a strong theme of communications running through all the stations.

The combined experience of consultants, registrars and junior doctors to write, edit and quality check these stations, promises to deliver content that is appropriate to reach a standard we would expect of new junior doctors entering their foundation internship years and into core training. It is important to know that these stations are all newly written and based at the level of clinical competencies we would expect from these grades of doctors. Learning objectives exist for undergraduate curricula and for the foundation years, and the scenarios are based and written around these. What they are not, are scenarios that have been 'borrowed' from any medical school.

Preparation is the key to success in most things, but never more so than for the OSCEs and a candidate that hasn't practised will soon be found out. These books will allow you to practice relevant scenarios with verified checklists to learn both content and the generic approach. The format will allow you to practice in groups with one person being the candidate, one the actor and one the examiner. Each scenario finishes with three learning points. Picture these as are three core learning tips that we would want you to take away if you had only a couple of days left to the exam. These OSCE scenarios promise to be a robust revision aide for the student looking to recap and consolidate for their exams, but equally importantly prepare them for life in clinical practice.

I am immensely proud of this OSCESmart series. I have had the pleasure of working with some of the brightest and most dynamic young clinicians and educators I know, and I am sure you will find this series covering the essential clinical specialties a truly robust and invaluable companion in those stressful times of revision. I must take this opportunity to thank my colleagues for all their hard work but most of all to thank my wonderful wife Molly for her unerring love and support and my sons Reuben and Rafael for all the joy they bring me.

Despite the challenging times the health service finds itself in, being a doctor remains a huge privilege. We hope that this OSCESmart series goes some way to help you achieve the excellence you and your patients deserve.
Best of luck, Dr Sam Thenabadu, 2016

# Introduction to OSCE Smart in Anaesthetics

With little more than a few days exposure to Anaesthetics and Critical Care at Medical School, many students find this strange world of new drugs, gases, vapours and equipment to be almost impenetrable. When the time comes for exam preparation, this can make it difficult to know where to begin. This book is designed to cover a broad base of core knowledge and skills that will be useful not only in your exam preparation, but also as you begin your career as a Foundation Doctor. It could also be used in preparation for Core Training interviews for Anaesthesia or Acute Care Common Stem.

We present a range of scenarios in Anaesthesia, Critical Care and Pain, demonstrating the breadth and variety of clinical experience you could expect from a career in Anaesthetics, from the Operating Theatre to the Labour Ward, ICU and the Emergency Department.

Our section on Preoperative Assessment will allow you to practice taking an Anaesthetic history and tailor your questioning to the particular challenges each patient may present to the Anaesthetist. These scenarios provide useful examples of how a patient's comorbidities can impact on the safe delivery of Anaesthesia. It should be clear that Anaesthetists need a solid grounding in General Medicine in order to evaluate and care for their patient's effectively. There are also more challenging scenarios dealing with specific Anaesthetic considerations like a patient with a known difficult airway or susceptibility to Malignant Hyperpyrexia.

There is a comprehensive section on Critical Care scenarios, dealing with a range of common emergency presentations. Here we look at them from the Anaesthetist's perspective, but the benefits of managing any medical emergency as part of a multidisciplinary team cannot be understated. We emphasise the importance of a thorough A-E assessment and calling for help as the cornerstones of safe acute care.

The theme of clear communication runs throughout the book, reflecting its central importance in the clinical environment. In particular there are stations testing your ability to break bad news with clarity and empathy and others requiring you to convey complex technical information in an understandable way. We cover data analysis relevant to the Anaesthetist, including arterial blood gases, ECG and Chest X-ray interpretation. In all these things, we must remain thorough and systematic in our approach. Time pressure and fatigue are unavoidable in our careers, but maintaining meticulous standards will help us to avoid errors that could cause harm to our patients.

I hope you will find this book useful in your exam preparation and I would like to wish you the very best of luck with your training and your future career. A big thank you to my Co-Authors for their hard work and dedication to this project, without whom none of this would have been possible. Not forgetting Sam Thenabadu, who is a friend and an inspiration.

**Dr Joe Lipton**

# About the Authors


## Dr Joe Lipton
### BSc MBBS MRCP FRCA

Anaesthetic Specialty Registrar, ST5, South London School of Anaesthesia


Joe Lipton is an Anaesthetic Registrar based in South East London. Having graduated from University College, London with 1st Class Honours in Psychology, Joe completed the 4 year graduate entry medical program at King's College London School of Medicine in 2008. He pursued his interest in Anaesthetics and Critical Care, initially via the Acute Care Common Stem Core Training pathway, before taking up a Specialist Training post in Anaesthetics based at Guy's & St Thomas' NHS Foundation trust.

His career interests include Cardiothoracic Anaesthesia and Medical Education and he has written and presented work at several national level education conferences. He has regular commitments as a Simulation Facilitator and Advanced Life Support Instructor and has been recognised for his contribution to Medical Education with a South Thames Foundation School Merit Award.

Joe is a father of two boys and has therefore had to remove the hobbies and interests section of this biography!

## Dr Sam Thenabadu
### MBBS MRCP DRCOG DCH MA Clin Ed FRCEM MSc (Paed) FHEA

Consultant Adult & Paediatric Emergency Medicine
Honorary Senior Lecturer & Associate Director of Medical Education

Sam Thenabadu graduated from King's College Medical School in 2001 and dual trained in Adult and Paediatric Emergency Medicine in London before being appointed a consultant in 2011 at the Princess Royal University Hospital. He has Masters degrees in Clinical Medical Education and Advanced Paediatrics.

He is undergraduate director of medical education at the King's College NHS Trust and the academic block lead for Emergency Medicine and Critical Care at King's College School of Medicine. At postgraduate level he has been the Pan London Health Education England lead for CT3 paediatric emergency medicine trainees since 2011. Academically he has previously written two textbooks and has published in peer review journals and given numerous oral and poster presentations at national conferences in emergency medicine, paediatrics, medical education and patient quality and safety.

He has an unashamed passion for medical education and strives to achieve excellence for himself, his colleagues and his patients, hoping to always deliver this through an enjoyable learning environment. Service delivery and educational need not be two separate entities, and he hopes that those who have had great teachers will take it upon themselves to do the same for others in the future.

**Co-Authors**

Dr Joe Lipton
BSc (Hons) MBBS MRCP FRCA
Speciality Registrar ST5, Anaesthetics
South London School of Anaesthesia

Dr Sarah Jane Muldoon
MBChB MRCP FRCA
Speciality Registrar ST5, Anaesthetics
South London School of Anaesthesia

Dr Michael Shaw
MBChB FRCA EDIC
Speciality Registrar ST7, Anaesthetics
South London School of Anaesthesia

Dr Toby Winterbottom
MBBS BSc (Hons) MRCEM FRCA
Speciality Registrar ST5, Anaesthetics
Kent, Surrey & Sussex School of Anaesthesia

Dr Folasade Onakoya
BSc (Hons) MBBS

Dr Marilyn Boampomaa
MBBS BSc (Hons)
Junior Clinical Fellow, Anaesthetics
Princess Alexandra Hospital

With original illustrations by Anushka Athique

**Abbreviations**

AAA – Abdominal aorta aneurysm
ABCDE – Airway, Breathing, Circulation, Disability, Exposure
ATLS – Advance Trauma Life Support
BD – Twice a day
BPH - Benign Prostatic Hyperplasia
BPM – Beats Per Minute
C-Spine – Cervical Spine
CT - Computerised tomography
CT IVU - Computerised tomography intravenous urogram
CXR – Chest Radiograph
DNAR - Do Not Attempt Resuscitation
DRE – Digital Rectal Examination
ERCP - Endoscopic Retrograde cholangiopancreatography
FNA- Fine Needle Aspiration
GORD - Gastro-oesophageal reflux disease
GP - General practitioner
ITU – Intensive Care Unit
IHD – Ischemic Heart Disease
MRCP - Magnetic resonance cholangiopancreatography
RUQ- Right upper quadrant
OD – Once a day
OSCEs - objective structured clinical examinations
PCA – Pain Control Analgesia
PRN- As when Required
PSA – Prostate-specific antigen
P-POSSUM – risk calculation in a preoperative patient
SOCRATES - mnemonic acronym used evaluate the nature of pain
TIA- Transient Ischemic Attack
USS - Ultrasound

# ANAESTHETIC PRE-ASSESSMENT OSCE – Known History of Difficult Airway

## Candidate's Instructions:

Martin Williams is a 52-year-old man who has presented for elective laparoscopic inguinal hernia repair under general anaesthetic.

You are a Foundation Year doctor on your Anaesthetic rotation and you have been asked to take a short history and perform an anaesthetic pre-assessment.

After 6 minutes the examiner will stop you and ask you to summarise back your findings and suggest your management plan.

## Examiner's Instructions:

Martin is a 52-year-old man who has presented for elective laparoscopic inguinal hernia repair under general anaesthetic.

He is an obese gentleman, body weight 115kg, height 182cm (BMI 34), who takes Ramipril 5mg for hypertension.

He had an anaesthetic 5 years ago for a cholecystectomy, and was told after the operation that there had been a problem putting a tube into his airway. He doesn't remember much more detail, but says his throat was very sore afterwards.

After six minutes, ask the candidate to summarise the case and suggest what they would do next. Can they suggest a safe plan for providing anaesthesia?

## Actor's Instructions:

You are a 52-year-old man and are expecting to have keyhole surgery today to repair an inguinal hernia in your right groin.

You are worried about your operation, and are keen to speak to an anaesthetist. 5 years ago you had key-hole surgery in this same hospital to have your gallbladder removed, and when you woke up afterwards you had a very sore throat and were told it had been difficult to insert a breathing tube. You were kept in hospital overnight for observation, but allowed home the next day. If asked, you were not admitted to ICU.

You are hoping to be reassured that this won't happen again today, and even wonder if you can avoid a general anaesthetic all together. You will be satisfied if the doctor explains that they will get a more senior colleague to speak with you about different methods of securing a breathing tube, or performing a spinal anaesthetic instead.

The doctor taking your history may ask you to open your mouth or make other simple facial expressions. If you are asked if you have any dental work, you will report that you have two crowns on your upper incisors.

You know you have put on weight since your last anaesthetic, and volunteer that you are a bit embarrassed that the admission nurse has documented your BMI as 34. If asked, you report that you take Ramipril 5mg a day for high blood pressure, smoke 10 cigarettes a day and drink 3-4 pints in the pub on a Friday. You are not allergic to anything.

**ANAESTHETIC PRE-ASSESSMENT OSCE - Known History of Difficult Airway**

| Task: | Achieved | Not Achieved |
|---|---|---|
| Introduces self & establishes rapport | | |
| Clarifies planned procedure and indication | | |
| Asks about previous anaesthetics | | |
| Takes a medical history – cardiovascular/ respiratory/ systemic enquiry | | |
| Asks about cardio-respiratory fitness/exercise tolerance | | |
| Asks about acid reflux | | |
| Asks about fasting status (solids & liquids) | | |
| Takes a drug history including allergies | | |
| Takes a social history (smoking/alcohol/illegal drugs) | | |
| Takes a family history (including problems with general anaesthesia) | | |
| Clarifies details of previous anaesthetic – was operation completed successfully, was patient woken up before surgery started, any awake fibreoptic intubation or tracheostomy, was he admitted to ICU? | | |
| Seeks signs/symptoms suggestive of Obstructive Sleep Apnea – snoring, apneas, somnolence, obesity, hypertension. | | |
| Performs a basic airway assessment (mouth opening/mallampati score/neck movement) | | |
| Assesses dentition/asks about caps, crowns or implants | | |
| Addresses patients concerns/answers questions | | |
| Explains concerns about possible risks of general anaesthetic in understandable language | | |
| Summarises case to examiner | | |
| Identifies past history of difficult intubation | | |
| Identifies need to discuss with senior and obtain previous anaesthetic chart | | |
| Can suggest awake fibreoptic intubation and/or avoiding GA entirely by using a neuroaxial/regional technique. | | |
| Examiner's Global Mark | /5 | |
| Actor / Helper's Global Mark | /5 | |
| Total Station Mark | /30 | |

## Learning Points

- The incidence of "failed intubation" is quoted as 1 in 1-2000 anaesthetics, and the more serious situation of "can't intubate can't ventilate" occurs in fewer than 1 in 5000 anaesthetics.

- The ability to provide oxygen is far more important than being able to place an endotracheal tube, so an assessment of how easy it will be to ventilate the patient with a bag and mask is as important as assessing the likely ease of intubation.

- If a patient is known to be a difficult intubation, the surgery could be performed, if appropriate, under spinal anaesthetic or regional nerve block. Alternatively, if an endotracheal tube is required it could be placed while the patient is still awake using a fibreoptic endoscope – Awake Fibreoptic Intubation.

# ANAESTHETIC PRE-ASSESSMENT OSCE - Patient with diabetes

## Candidate's Instructions:

Steve is a 54-year-old man who has presented to the pre-assessment clinic for a planned elective shoulder arthroscopy under general anaesthetic.

You are a Foundation Year1 doctor on your Anaesthetics rotation and you have been asked to perform an Anaesthetic pre-assessment.

After 6 minutes the examiner will stop you and ask you to summarise back your findings and suggest your management plan.

## Examiner's Instructions:

Steve is a 54-year-old male who has presented for an elective shoulder arthroscopy under general anaesthetic.

He has a past medical history of type II diabetes, which was diagnosed by his GP 7 years ago. He has found it difficult to control his blood sugars and was started on basal bolus insulin therapy by his diabetologist earlier this year. Despite this he regularly finds his blood sugars rise above 10mmol/L after meals, despite good treatment compliance.

In addition he has been diagnosed with hypertension for which he takes ramipril and amlodipine. At his last retinal screening he was told he has some early changes of retinopathy and is having annual surveillance for this. He has also been told that his kidney function is mildly impaired. He sees a podiatrist regularly and has no problems with foot ulcers or peripheral neuropathy.

He has no past history of ischaemic heart disease or stroke and is a non-smoker. He tries to take regular exercise and can easily climb a flight of stairs.

He had a general anaesthetic 4 years ago for incision and drainage of a groin abscess which was uneventful. He suffers with severe reflux for which he takes omeprazole. He has no loose teeth and no risk factors for a difficult airway.

The candidate will be expected to take a thorough past medical history including of the patient's diabetes related complications. They will need to answer the patient's questions about perioperative fasting and give sensible advice about how to manage his insulin therapy.

After six minutes ask the candidate to summarise back and then ask the significance of severe gastro-oesophageal reflux for the conduct of Anaesthesia and how this impacts on airway management.

## Actor's Instructions:

You are Steve, a 54-year-old man presenting to the pre-assessment clinic in preparation for shoulder surgery. You injured your shoulder playing rugby some years ago and it has become increasingly stiff and painful over the last few years.

You consider yourself to be in reasonable health, although you have type II diabetes for which you are taking insulin. You try to be very careful about what you eat and check your blood sugars regularly throughout the day. Despite this you sometimes find your sugars difficult to control and regularly get readings of over 10 after meals. At the moment you are taking lantus 10 units at night and 8 units of novorapid with your meals.

You have your diabetes managed in the diabetes clinic where you have regular eye screening, foot care and blood tests. You are aware that there are some early diabetes related changes at the back of your eyes and that your kidney function is mildly impaired. You've never had a problem with your feet and don't suffer with any numbness.

You take amlodipine and ramipril for your blood pressure which you believe is well controlled. Of late you have been suffering with a lot of heartburn for which you have started taking omeprazole. You get burning in the back of your throat after most meals and sometimes stomach contents comes up into your mouth when lying in bed a night.

You had a general anaesthetic 4 years ago for incision and drainage of an abscess which was uneventful. You have no loose teeth, caps, crowns or dentures.

You are concerned about how to manage your blood sugars around the time of surgery and would like some advice about which medicines you should or shouldn't take.

ANAESTHETIC PRE-ASSESSMENT OSCE - Patient with diabetes

| Task: | Achieved | Not Achieved |
|---|---|---|
| Introduces self & establishes rapport | | |
| Clarifies planned procedure and indication | | |
| Asks about previous anaesthetics | | |
| Takes a medical history – cardiovascular/respiratory/systemic enquiry | | |
| Establishes diagnosis of type II diabetes | | |
| Asks about treatment for diabetes | | |
| Asks about glycaemic control | | |
| Asks about macrovascular complications (ischaemic heart disease/stroke) | | |
| Asks about microvascular/other complications (retinopathy/nephropathy/neuropathy) | | |
| Asks about cardiorespiratory fitness/exercise tolerance | | |
| Asks about smoking and alcohol consumption | | |
| Establishes presence of severe reflux | | |
| Performs a basic airway assessment (mouth opening/mallampati score/neck movement) | | |
| Assesses dentition/asks about caps, crowns or implants | | |
| Addresses patients concerns about medications around time of surgery | | |
| Advises to take long acting insulin as normal the night before surgery and omit short acting insulin on the day of surgery | | |
| Reassures patient that blood sugars will be measured regularly and controlled during the periopertive period | | |
| Summarises case to examiner | | |
| Aware that severe reflux increases risk of aspiration of gastric contents | | |
| Knows aspiration risk mandates insertion of a definitive airway/rapid sequence induction | | |
| | | |
| Examiner's Global Mark | /5 | |
| Actor / Helper's Global Mark | /5 | |
| Total Station Mark | /30 | |

## Learning Points

- Diabetes affects 10-15% of the adult surgical population and patients with diabetes have higher rates of complications, mortality and length of hospital stay.

- In order to minimise glycaemic complications for diabetic patients undergoing surgery, it is important that the peri-operative fasting time is kept to a minimum. This can be achieved by ensuring diabetic patients are scheduled first on the operating list. A blood sugar target of 6-10mmol/L is recommended. Patients undergoing long procedures with multiple missed doses of their usual treatment should be managed with a 'variable rate intravenous insulin infusion' (formerly known as an insulin sliding scale).

- Poorly controlled diabetes can be associated with gastro-oesophageal reflux, sometimes related to autonomic neuropathy causing impaired gastric emptying. Patients who are severely symptomatic with reflux are treated in the same way as those who have a full stomach. This means performing a rapid sequence induction of Anaesthesia with insertion of a cuffed endotracheal tube - a 'definitive airway'.

# ANAESTHETIC PRE-ASSESSMENT OSCE - Obesity and sequelae

## Candidate's Instructions:

Oliver is a 52-year-old man presenting for an elective umbilical hernia repair under general anaesthetic.

You are a Foundation Year1 doctor on your anaesthetics rotation and you have been asked to perform an Anaesthetic pre-assessment.

After 6 minutes the examiner will stop you and ask you to summarise back your findings and suggest your management plan.

## Examiner's Instructions:

Oliver is a 52-year-old patient who has presented for a repair of umbilical hernia under general anaesthetic. His anaesthetic history is unremarkable.

He is obese, with a body weight of 120kg, height of 1.73m and a BMI of 40 kg/$m^2$.

In addition to obesity Oliver is treated for hypercholesterolaemia, and hypertension. He displays elements of obstructive sleep apnoea (OSA), namely daytime somnolence and snoring, and has a large collar size (>17 inches / 43cm).

After the candidate has taken the history, ask them to summarise the case and say how they would proceed next. One aspect of this station is knowledge of the Body Mass Index (BMI) and its calculation; the candidate should be asked how they would calculate BMI (BMI = mass in kg / height in $metres^2$).

These patients represent a high risk of airway compromise in the peri-operative period, particularly after general anaesthetic. The candidate should offer that they would consult with a senior anaesthetic colleague, and give some consideration to the appropriate area for post-operative care (high-dependency unit).

After six minutes ask the candidate to summarise back and then ask directly about the best place for post operative care and how to calculate the BMI.

## Actor's Instructions:

You are a 52-year-old man who has had an umbilical hernia for many years, which is now bothering you and has become painful at times. You definitely want to proceed with your operation today.

You had a general anaesthetic as a 5-year-old to have your tonsils removed, with no problems. Family members have had anaesthetics with no concerns.

Your work as a taxi driver means you keep irregular hours, with little exercise and a poor diet. You have put on weight over the last 2 years and weigh around 20 stone. Your GP has started you on tablets for high blood pressure and high cholesterol in that time. These are well controlled at the moment, and you've never had any heart problems. You don't smoke or drink alcohol, and you have no allergies.

If asked you should offer that you have a big collar size (18 inches), your wife often comments on your loud snoring, and you are often feel tired in the daytime, even if you haven't worked late shifts. If the candidate doesn't specifically ask about these factors related to obesity then volunteer that you are aware you are overweight and would like to know if this will affect the anaesthetic.

**ANAESTHETIC PRE-ASSESSMENT OSCE - Obesity and sequelae**

| Task: | Achieved | Not Achieved |
|---|---|---|
| Introduces self & establishes rapport | | |
| Clarifies planned procedure and indication | | |
| Asks about previous anaesthetics | | |
| Takes a medical history – cardiovascular/respiratory/systemic enquiry | | |
| Clarifies current weight / height / BMI | | |
| Takes a drug history including allergies | | |
| Elicits history of daytime somnolence, snoring | | |
| Asks about collar size | | |
| Asks about cardio-respiratory fitness/exercise tolerance | | |
| Asks about acid reflux | | |
| Asks about fasting status (solids & liquids) | | |
| Takes a social history (smoking/alcohol/illegal drugs) | | |
| Takes a family history (including problems with general anaesthesia) | | |
| Performs a basic airway assessment (mouth opening/mallampati score/neck movement) | | |
| Assesses dentition/asks about caps, crowns or implants | | |
| Addresses patients concerns/answers questions | | |
| Explains concerns about possible risks of general anaesthetic in understandable language | | |
| Summarises case to examiner | | |
| Indicates may require care in high-dependency-unit (HDU) post-operatively | | |
| Can describe how to calculate BMI when asked | | |
| | | |
| Examiner's Global Mark | /5 | |
| Actor / Helper's Global Mark | /5 | |
| Total Station Mark | /30 | |

## Learning Points

- Obesity – defined as a body mass index (BMI) greater than $30kg/m^2$ – is becoming increasingly prevalent in the healthcare setting. At present around 25% of the UK adult population are classed as obese, with this number predicted to reach at least 50% by 2050.

- Obese patients have a higher risk of a range of systemic diseases (including hypertension, ischaemic heart disease, airways disease, and diabetes mellitus) and a higher risk of mortality compared to non-obese patients.

- Obese patients with obstructive sleep apnoea (OSA) are of particular relevance to anaesthetists, as symptoms of airway obstruction and hypoxia can be worsened after general anaesthesia. The STOP BANG questionnaire can be used to screen for the likelihood of OSA, and includes assessment of snoring, tiredness and neck circumference alongside other patient factors. Patients with OSA may require HDU care post-operatively.

# ANAESTHETIC PRE-ASSESSMENT OSCE - Family history of Malignant Hyperpyrexia

## Candidate's Instructions:

Ian is a 28-year-old man who has presented for elective excision of a lipoma under general anaesthetic.

You are a Foundation doctor on your anaesthetics rotation and you have been asked to perform an Anaesthetic pre-assessment.

After 6 minutes the examiner will stop you and ask you to summarise back your findings and suggest your management plan.

## Examiner's Instructions:

Ian is a 28-year-old male who has presented for elective excision of a lipoma under general anaesthetic.

He is fit and healthy and has no medical problems. He has a family history consistent with possible susceptibility to Malignant Hyperpyrexia – his father having been admitted to intensive care following a general anaesthetic some years previously.

After six minutes ask the candidate to summarise the case and say how they would proceed next. Ask them which types of anaesthetic drugs can trigger malignant hyperpyrexia.

## Actor's Instructions:

You are a 28-year-old man presenting for surgery to remove a lipoma on your back that has been bothering you for a while. You are hoping to have it removed before going away on a beach holiday with your new girlfriend this summer.

You are fit and healthy and have no medical problems. You take no regular medications and have no allergies that you know of. You don't smoke and drink occasionally with friends, but not excessively.

You remember being told by your mother that your father had suffered a reaction to an anaesthetic some years before. His body temperature had risen very high and his operation had to be abandoned. He had to go to intensive care and was very ill for several days, but made a full recovery. After that you think that the family were tested to see whether what happened to your dad might run in the family. You don't know what the results of these tests were and you are no longer in contact with your parents after a family dispute.

You are very keen to have your operation today and will try to persuade the doctor taking your history that you'll be fine with the anaesthetic. After they explain the possible risks, you are happy to wait and see the Consultant Anaesthetist to talk further about your anaesthetic.

**ANAESTHETIC PRE-ASSESSMENT OSCE - Family history of Malignant Hyperpyrexia**

| Task: | Achieved | Not Achieved |
|---|---|---|
| Introduces self & establishes rapport | | |
| Clarifies planned procedure and indication | | |
| Asks about previous anaesthetics | | |
| Takes a medical history – cardiovascular/respiratory/systemic enquiry | | |
| Asks about cardio-respiratory fitness/exercise tolerance | | |
| Asks about acid reflux | | |
| Takes a drug history including allergies | | |
| Takes a social history (smoking/alcohol/illegal drugs) | | |
| Takes a family history (including problems with general anaesthesia) | | |
| Clarifies details of family history (father's ICU admission/high body temperature) | | |
| Asks about family testing for MH | | |
| Asks about fasting status (solids & liquids) | | |
| Performs a basic airway assessment (mouth opening/mallampati score/neck movement) | | |
| Assesses dentition/asks about caps, crowns or implants | | |
| Addresses patients concerns/answers questions | | |
| Explains concerns about possible risks of general anaesthetic in understandable language | | |
| Summarises case to examiner | | |
| Identifies possible susceptibility to Malignant Hyperpyrexia | | |
| Identifies need to discuss with senior and possibly postpone operation | | |
| Can identify volatile anaesthetic agents and muscle relaxants as MH triggers | | |
| | | |
| Examiner's Global Mark | /5 | |
| Actor / Helper's Global Mark | /5 | |
| Total Station Mark | /30 | |

## Learning Points

- Malignant Hyperpyrexia (MH) is a rare, but life threatening condition which occurs when susceptible individuals are exposed to volatile anaesthetic agents (e.g. sevoflurane) or the muscle relaxant suxamethonium.

- MH is a clinical diagnosis made during the perioperative period after exposure to triggering agents causes a rise in core body temperature (>40 degrees C), increased CO2 production, acidosis and muscle breakdown.

- Affected individuals and their families are referred to Malignant Hyperthermia Units ( in the UK this is based at St James' Hospital in Leeds) where they undergo diagnostic testing for condition through DNA analysis and muscle biopsy.

# ANAESTHETIC PRE-ASSESSMENT OSCE - Patient with ischaemic heart disease presenting for elective surgery

## Candidate's Instructions:

John is a 78-year-old man who has presented for elective inguinal hernia repair under general anaesthetic.

You are a Foundation Year1 doctor on your anaesthetics rotation and you have been asked to perform an Anaesthetic pre-assessment, including answering any questions he may have.

After 6 minutes the examiner will stop you and ask you to summarise back your findings and suggest your management plan and answer some brief questions.

## Examiner's Instructions:

John is a 78-year-old male who has presented for elective inguinal hernia repair under general anaesthetic.

He has a history of cardiac disease and suffered a myocardial infarction 2 years ago. He has two coronary stents and is currently asymptomatic. He can climb two flights of stairs, walks 2 miles every day and lives independently at home. He has no signs or symptoms of cardiac failure. His baseline blood pressure is 145/70 and his oxygen saturations are normal.

After six minutes ask the candidate to summarise the case and the important issues. Ask them to comment on his risk and fitness for general anaesthesia and what further investigations they would like to review before his operation. Ask them then how the situation would be different if the patient had recently started to complain of worsening chest pain and shortness of breath.

## Actor's Instructions:

You are a 78-year-old man presenting for surgery to repair an inguinal hernia that has been causing pain.

You have previously had heart trouble and had a heart attack two years ago after which you had two stents inserted into the arteries supplying your heart. Following this you recovered well and currently live alone in a house with stairs and take your dog walking for a couple of miles each morning. You sleep with one pillow, don't have swollen ankles and have no other medical problems. You were last seen in the cardiology clinic around 6 months ago and were discharged back to primary care. Your last echo around this time was 'fine'.

You have no known respiratory disease, diabetes or stroke.

You had a general anaesthetic in 2000 for a knee replacement and had no problems.

You currently take a beta blocker, aspirin, a statin and ramipril. You have no allergies. You don't smoke and drink very occasionally at bridge club.

You are a little worried as you have heard having a general anaesthetic is very dangerous for someone who has had heart trouble. You feel quite fit but you would like to make sure everything has been done and no further tests are required. Speaking to a consultant anaesthetist would help allay your fears.

**ANAESTHETIC PRE-ASSESSMENT OSCE - Patient with ischaemic heart disease presenting for elective surgery**

| Task: | Achieved | Not Achieved |
|---|---|---|
| Introduces self & establishes rapport | | |
| Clarifies planned procedure | | |
| Asks about previous anaesthetics | | |
| Takes a medical history – cardiovascular/respiratory/systemic enquiry | | |
| Elicits history of myocardial infarction and 2 coronary stents | | |
| Asks about cardio-respiratory fitness/exercise tolerance | | |
| Asks about recent follow up/investigations | | |
| Asks about palpitations/loss of consciousness | | |
| Asks about signs of cardiac failure | | |
| Takes a drug history including allergies | | |
| Takes a social history (smoking/alcohol) | | |
| Performs a basic airway assessment (mouth opening/mallampati score/neck movement) | | |
| Explains concerns about mildly elevated risks of general anaesthetic for patients with stable, optimised cardiac disease | | |
| Addresses patients concerns/answers questions and offers a consultation with a senior anaesthetist | | |
| Summarises case to examiner | | |
| Identifies clinical picture of stable, optimised ischaemic heart disease | | |
| Asks to see baseline observations | | |
| Asks for a full blood count and U+E analysis | | |
| Asks to see a recent ECG | | |
| Knows that elective surgery should be postponed if patient has new/worsening angina | | |
| Examiner's Global Mark | /5 | |
| Actor / Helper's Global Mark | /5 | |
| Total Station Mark | /30 | |

## Learning Points

- Ischaemic heart disease is a risk factor for complications during and after general anaesthesia. Cardiac conditions that are associated with the highest perioperative risk are:

  Acute cardiac failure
  Recent MI (<30 days ago)
  Unstable angina
  Arrhythmia
  Symptomatic valvular disease

- As well as patient factors, the perioperative risk is also related to the type of surgical procedure. High risk surgeries include supra-inguinal vascular, intra-thoracic and intra-abdominal procedures.

- Asking about exercise tolerance is an extremely important screening tool. When trying to quantify a patient's perioperative risk, we usually express exercise tolerance in terms of 'metabolic equivalents' - or MET. 1 MET is defined as the oxygen consumption required to sit at rest in a chair. 4 MET is equivalent to climbing a flight of stairs and strenuous exercise is >10 MET. There is extensive evidence that an exercise tolerance of >4 MET indicates sufficient cardiorespiratory reserve to tolerate the physiological insult of undergoing general anaesthesia.

# ANAESTHETIC PRE-ASSESSMENT OSCE -

# Asthma with sensitivity to NSAIDs

## Candidate's Instructions:

Rachel is a 44-year-old woman presenting for an elective excision of a benign breast lump under general anaesthetic.

You are a Foundation Year1 doctor on your anaesthetics rotation and you have been asked to perform an Anaesthetic pre-assessment.

After 6 minutes the examiner will stop you and ask you to summarise back your findings and suggest your management plan.

## Examiner's Instructions:

Rachel is a 44-year-old patient who has presented for an excision of a benign breast lump under general anaesthetic.

She has had a previous general anaesthetic for an appendicectomy twenty years ago, which was uneventful.

Significantly, she suffers from asthma. She has had multiple Emergency Department admissions with acute asthma attacks, and three years ago had an admission to ICU after use of diclofenac led to a life-threatening exacerbation of her asthma. She was intubated and ventilated for 48 hours on that occasion.

Currently her asthma is well controlled using inhalers and oral montelukast. Otherwise she has no long-term medical problems, and is a lifelong non-smoker.

After six minutes ask the candidate to summarise the case and say how they would proceed. Ask them if there are any further investigations they would request prior to general anaesthetic.

## Actor's Instructions:

You are a 44-year-old woman who has had a breast lump that you noticed 6 months ago. The hospital has performed a needle biopsy under local anaesthetic and you have been assured the lump is benign. The surgeons have recommended removal for more formal testing and peace of mind, and you are attending today for the operation under general anaesthetic.

You have had a general anaesthetic in the past for an appendix operation and had no problems.

You have been treated for asthma since you were a child, and are known to the respiratory team in the hospital, seeing them every 6 months or so. At your last appointment the consultant added in a tablet medication to help control symptoms. You use a purple inhaler (Seretide) twice daily, and a blue inhaler (Ventolin) when required. You also take a tablet (montelukast) once daily. This allows you to continue exercise regularly. You have never smoked.

You have been to the Emergency Department multiple times because of asthma attacks, and on one occasion had an admission to the Intensive Care Unit (ICU) after a reaction to a pain medication. After using diclofenac for an ankle injury your wheeze came on severely and you required 2 days on a ventilator. It was a very scary experience for you, and you are very worried about these types of drugs (NSAIDs) and need reassurance they won't be used. You want to make sure the allergy is recorded on your notes. As long as you can be reassured you will be happy to continue to general anesthetic.

**ANAESTHETIC PRE-ASSESSMENT OSCE - Asthma with sensitivity to NSAIDs**

| Task: | Achieved | Not Achieved |
|---|---|---|
| Introduces self & establishes rapport | | |
| Clarifies planned procedure and indication | | |
| Asks about previous anaesthetics | | |
| Takes a medical history – cardiovascular/respiratory/systemic enquiry | | |
| Clarifies specific asthma history regarding emergency and critical care admissions | | |
| Takes a drug history including allergies | | |
| Elicits history of life-threatening reaction to diclofenac | | |
| Asks about cardio-respiratory fitness/exercise tolerance | | |
| Asks about acid reflux | | |
| Asks about fasting status (solids & liquids) | | |
| Takes a social history (smoking/alcohol/illegal drugs) | | |
| Takes a family history (including problems with general anaesthesia) | | |
| Performs a basic airway assessment (mouth opening/mallampati score/neck movement) | | |
| Assesses dentition/asks about caps, crowns or implants | | |
| Addresses patients concerns/answers questions | | |
| Able to reassure patient NSAIDs are recorded as an allergy on the patient record | | |
| Explains concerns about possible risks of general anaesthetic in understandable language | | |
| Summarises case to examiner | | |
| Can identify other NSAID agents (e.g., ibuprofen, parecoxib) as potential triggers | | |
| Mentions use of peak flow measurement, pulse oximetry and chest radiograph as potential investigations | | |
| | | |
| Examiner's Global Mark | /5 | |
| Actor / Helper's Global Mark | /5 | |
| Total Station Mark | /30 | |

## Learning Points

- Up to 25% of individuals with asthma may suffer from NSAID-induced wheeze, it is essential to specifically enquire about previous NSAID usage in asthmatics.

- The British Thoracic Society produces guidelines for the step-wise pharmacological treatment for asthma. Treatment with oral bronchodilator agents (leukotriene antagonists such as montelukast or methylxanthines such as aminophylline) should alert you to those patients with more 'brittle' asthma.

- Multiple inhalers exist for patients with asthma and chronic obstructive pulmonary disease (COPD). It is helpful to learn which colour inhaler matches which therapy to aid you taking a drug history.

# DATA INTERPRETATION - ECG Interpretation

## Candidate's Instructions:

You are the Foundation Year1 on an anaesthetics rotation, and are attending the afternoon outpatient pre-assessment clinic with the consultant anaesthetist (who is yet to arrive). It is 2pm on the 13th June.

Andrew is a 59-year-old man listed for an inguinal hernia repair. He has a history of hypertension and diabetes. His diabetes and hypertension are poorly controlled.

He is presently experiencing some shortness of breath and chest tightness after rushing to get to the appointment on time. A 12-lead ECG has been performed by the pre-assessment nurses.

Make a brief assessment of the patient, review the ECG and explain your findings and plan to the patient. After six minutes the examiner will ask you to present your finding and to describe the ECG.

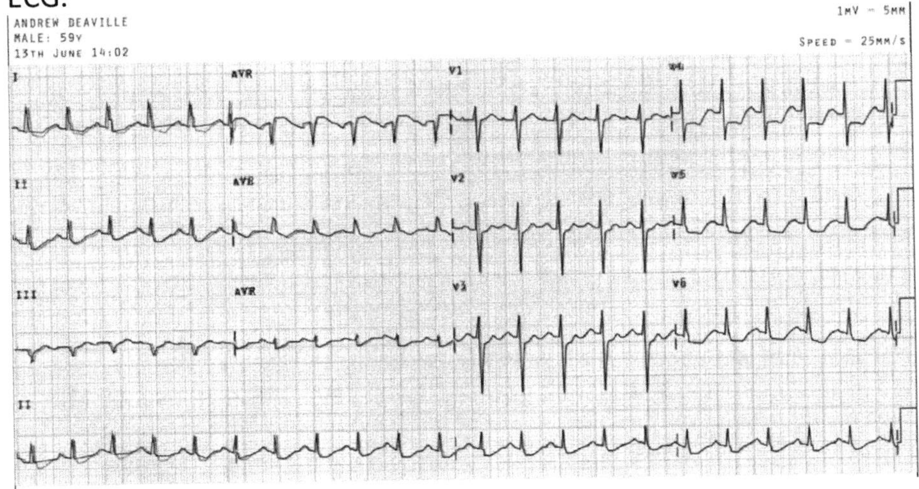

## Examiner's Instructions:

Andrew is a 59-year-old patient attending the outpatient pre-assessment anaesthetic clinic prior to an elective inguinal hernia repair. He has poorly controlled hypertension and diabetes, and is currently experiencing symptoms related to acute myocardial ischaemia having rushed to attend the appointment. He has never suffered angina or a myocardial infarction. In the context of his diabetes he is experiencing chest tightness and shortness of breath, without pain. He is treated regularly with amlodipine, ramipril, metformin simvastatin, and aspirin. He has no allergies. His previous ECG is completely normal.

The pre-assessment nurse has completed a 12-lead ECG and the candidate should be able to interpret this systematically. It reveals the following findings:

| | |
|---|---|
| Rate: | ~ 100 beats/min |
| Rhythm: | Sinus rhythm |
| Axis: | Normal axis |
| PR interval: | Normal (200 ms) |
| QRS duration: | Normal (120 ms) |
| QRS amplitude: | Normal |
| ST segment: | ST depression lead II, V4 – V6 |
| QT interval: | Normal |
| **Diagnosis:** | **Acute ischaemia (in lateral leads)** |

The patient's blood pressure is 145/90 and $SpO_2$ 96% on room air. Blood sugar is 7.5 mmol/L.

**The candidate should elicit the acute symptoms, and interpret the ECG. They should be directly asked elements of the mark scheme.** They should be asked about their immediate management of this patient. In this case the appropriate management would be to arrange an admission via the Emergency Department or the in-patient cardiology team, with consideration of oxygen, nitrate and analgesic therapy.

In light of the ECG findings it will be prudent to delay surgery until a full assessment and recommendations have been made by the cardiology team.

## Actor's Instructions:

You are a 59-year-old man attending the outpatient pre-assessment clinic prior to having your inguinal hernia repaired in 2 weeks' time. You had trouble parking and have rushed from the furthest car park to get to the clinic.

You feel unwell, and have chest tightness like a band around your chest. You feel a little out of breath. You don't have any pain, and there is no specific point in your chest that feels worse than any other. You haven't ever experienced this before, and are worried.

You do know that your GP has been concerned about your recent blood pressure control and has started ramipril alongside your other medications. Your diabetes is also very variable, and your GP has talked about starting another diabetic medicine alongside your metformin. You have never had angina or a heart attack, but your dad had a heart attack in his fifties.

The nurse has taken a heart trace, and the doctor will check this with you present. It reveals an abnormality that requires urgent assessment and treatment in the Emergency Department. You would like to know what the test shows. You feel reassured that the doctor is taking this seriously, and happy to do what they suggest. You would like to know whether this will delay your surgery.

**DATA INTERPRETATION - ECG Interpretation**

| Task: | Achieved | Not Achieved |
|---|---|---|
| Introduces self and establishes rapport | | |
| Elucidates past medical history / drugs / allergies | | |
| Elucidates current symptoms | | |
| Ensures ECG of relevant patient | | |
| Ensures ECG timed and dated correctly | | |
| Explains calculation of rate | | |
| Correct rate calculated (~100 beats/min) | | |
| Identifies rhythm (sinus rhythm) | | |
| Identifies axis (normal) | | |
| Explains reason for P wave (atrial depolarisation) | | |
| Explains reason for QRS complex (ventricular depolarisation) | | |
| Defines PR interval and normal duration (200 ms) | | |
| Defines QRS duration and normal value (120 ms) | | |
| Identifies ST segment depression (in leads V4 – V6) | | |
| Identifies ST changes likely due to ischaemia | | |
| Recognises significance of ECG changes in context of symptoms | | |
| States would refer to Emergency Department or cardiologists for further urgent assessment | | |
| Mentions assessment of vital signs (BP, $SpO_2$) | | |
| Mentions initial therapy (oxygen / nitrates / analgesia / aspirin) | | |
| Demonstrates calm, reassuring manner. Realistic regarding potential surgery delay | | |
| | | |
| Examiner's Global Mark | /5 | |
| Actor / Helper's Global Mark | /5 | |
| Total Station Mark | /30 | |

## Learning Points

- Ischaemic pain from the myocardium may present atypically in diabetic patients. A range of symptoms may be described including chest tightness, indigestion, nausea, belching and shortness of breath. Some patients may experience no symptoms ('silent ischaemia'), therefore a degree of clinical suspicion is required in patients with multiple risk factors.

- ECG interpretation is a key skill for every doctor. It is worthwhile developing and practicing a systematic approach to ensure consistent, thorough interpretation of any ECG. Practice using normal ECG traces allows the development of 'pattern recognition', making it easier to spot subtle abnormalities when they arise.

- Occasionally patients present with unanticipated acute problems through a non-acute route. It is important to know what the appropriate channels are to co-ordinate their care. It is not unheard for an ambulance to be called to move a patient from one area of the hospital to the Emergency Department. Patient safety must come first.

# DATA INTERPRETATION OSCE - Chest X-ray interpretation

## Candidate's Instructions:

You are the Foundation Doctor in ICU. You have been asked by one of the nursing students to help interpret a chest X-ray taken of Ray (Hospital Number AA123456) , a 57 year old man who was admitted to the unit with respiratory failure.

Please talk the nursing student through the systematic interpretation of a chest X-ray and answer any questions they may have.

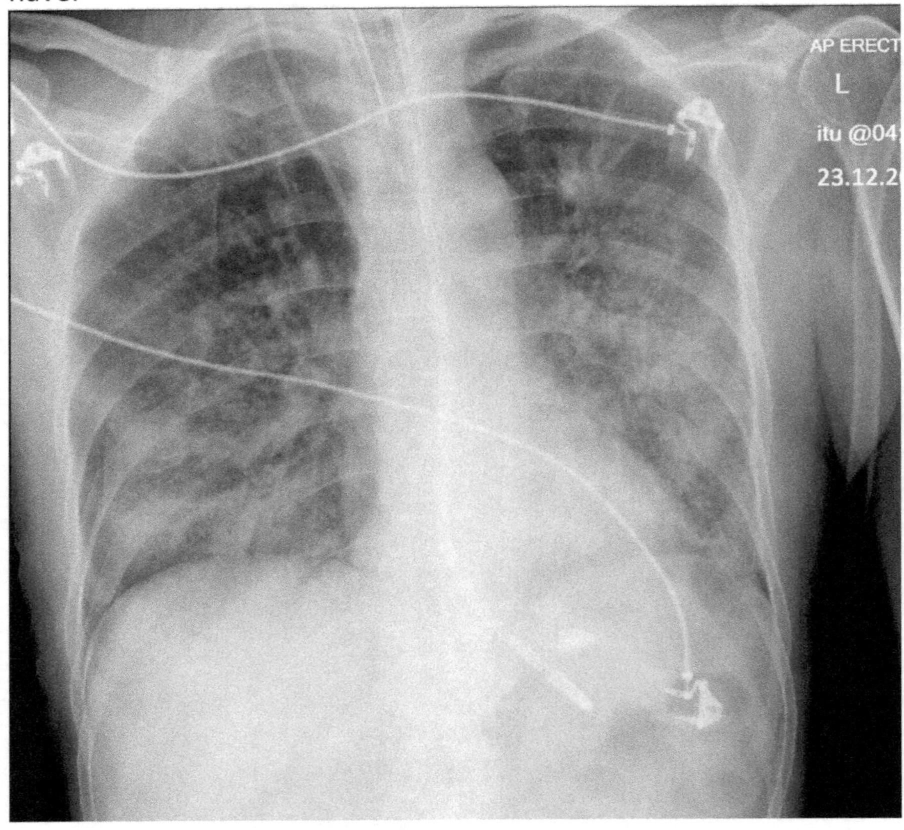

## Examiner's Instructions:

The candidate is a Foundation Year 1 Doctor working in the Intensive Care Unit. They have been asked by one the Nursing students in the unit to talk them through a chest X-ray belonging to one of the patients admitted with respiratory failure.

The candidate will be expected to demonstrate a methodical, systematic approach to chest X-ray interpretation, identifying the correct positioning of the endotracheal tube, central venous line and nasogastric tube. They should also recognise the features of consolidation.

In addition to their ability to comment accurately on the radiological features, you will also be assessing them on their communication with a junior Nursing colleague.

## Actor's Instructions:

You are a final year nursing student currently on placement in Intensive Care. The patient you are looking after, who was admitted with respiratory failure and is currently on a ventilator, had a chest X-ray taken overnight which you are keen to look at.

You have asked one of the Foundation Year doctors to talk you through the interpretation of a chest X-ray. In particular you are interested in how to confirm the correct position of the Nasogastric tube. On a previous placement there was a patient you were looking after who had an NG tube in the wrong place and received feed into their lung, making them very ill. You were told at the time that this was a 'never event', but you were not sure what this meant. Ask the doctor to explain the meaning of the term never event.

**DATA INTERPRETATION OSCE - Chest X-ray interpretation**

| Task: | Achieved | Not Achieved |
|---|---|---|
| Introduces self & establishes rapport | | |
| Checks nurses understanding/previous experience | | |
| Explains need for systematic approach to chest X-ray interpretation | | |
| Checks correct patient identification on X-ray | | |
| Checks time & date | | |
| Comments on AP projection | | |
| Comments on adequacy, penetration and exposure of film | | |
| Comments on rotation of film | | |
| Identifies presence of endotracheal tube | | |
| Comments on correct placement above carina | | |
| Comments on consolidation in lung fields | | |
| Comments on cardiac silhouette | | |
| Comments on hemidiaphragms/costophrenic angles | | |
| Notes presence of Right internal jugular central venous line | | |
| Comments on correct positioning in SVC/above right atrium | | |
| Comments on bony anatomy | | |
| Notes presence of nasogastric tube | | |
| Comments on correct position - descends in midline, ends below diaphragm in stomach | | |
| Gives correct definition of a never event | | |
| Uses understandable language and addresses nursing students learning needs | | |
| | | |
| Examiner's Global Mark | /5 | |
| Actor / Helper's Global Mark | /5 | |
| Total Station Mark | /30 | |

## Learning Points

- Interpretation of a chest X-ray must be done systematically, ideally using the same technique every single time. Relying on the 'quick eyeball' strategy will invariably lead to errors and you should resist the temptation to cut corners, however busy you are!

- Nasogastric tubes are inserted into most ICU patients and there must be a robust procedure in place to confirm their position. If possible, a gastric aspirate may be obtained and tested using pH indicator paper. A pH of <5.5 is considered acceptable. If it is not possible to aspirate anything from the tube or the pH is too high, then a chest X-ray is required to confirm correct placement in the stomach.

- 'Never events' are hot topics in the NHS. They are defined by NHS England as 'serious incidents that are wholly preventable as guidance or safety recommendations that provide strong systemic protective barriers are available at a national level and should have been implemented by all healthcare providers.' Examples relevant to Anaesthesia include wrong site surgery/regional Anaesthetic block and feeding in a misplaced NG tube.

# DATA INTERPRETATION OSCE – CAPNOGRAPHY WAVERFORM ANALYSIS

## Candidate's instructions:

You are a Foundation Year 1 doctor doing an anaesthetics rotation. A student Operating Department Practitioner (ODP) asks you for some help understanding Waveform Capnography.

Please explain to them why Waveform Capnography is used, then examine five diagrams from their textbook and explain the clinical significance of the various waveforms. Suggest what measures may need to be taken in clinical practice to identify or correct the problems leading to any abnormalities in each trace.

## Examiner's instructions

The candidate is to take the role of a Foundation Year doctor in Anaesthetics, teaching a student ODP about Waveform Capnography.

Present them with six Capnography waveforms.
Ask them to outline the reason capnography is used in clinical practice, and then explain each of the capnography traces to the student ODP, including any abnormalities, the clinical significance of these abnormalities, and what steps should be taken to further identify or treat the problem.

Waveform 1: Normal capnography trace.
Waveform 2: Trace suggesting obstruction to expiration.
Waveform 3: Trace suggesting sudden loss of cardiac output.
Waveform 4: Trace suggesting patient making respiratory effort against ventilator.
Waveform 5: Trace suggesting disconnection from breathing circuit.

## Actor's instructions

The candidate is to take the role of a Foundation Year1 in Anaesthetics, while you are a student ODP. You have asked the candidate to explain to you why Waveform Capnography is used, and to help you understand six different capnography waveforms.

After their initial explanation of capnography, show them each trace in turn. If prompting is required to move through the station, for each waveform ask;

What does this waveform show – is it abnormal?
What clinical problem(s) could produce this waveform?
What can we do to identify or correct the problem(s)?

If they are unable to complete a waveform, allow them to move onto the next.

# Capnography Waveforms

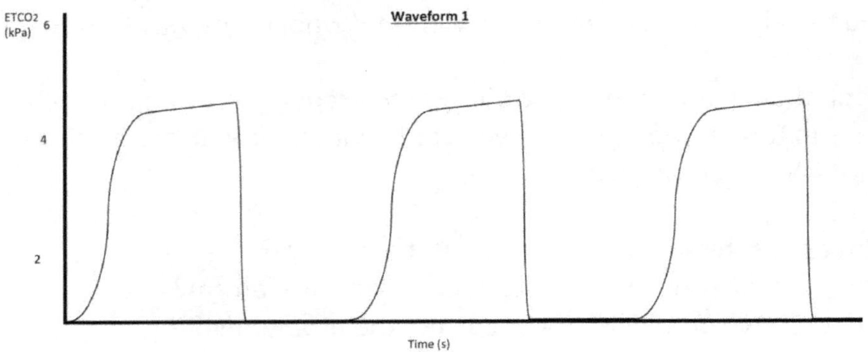


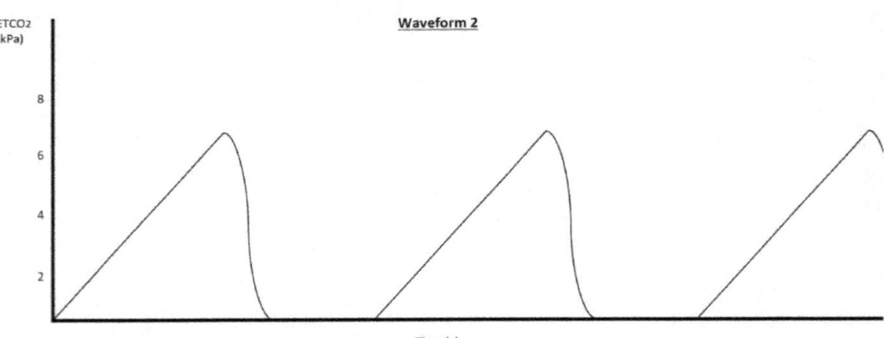

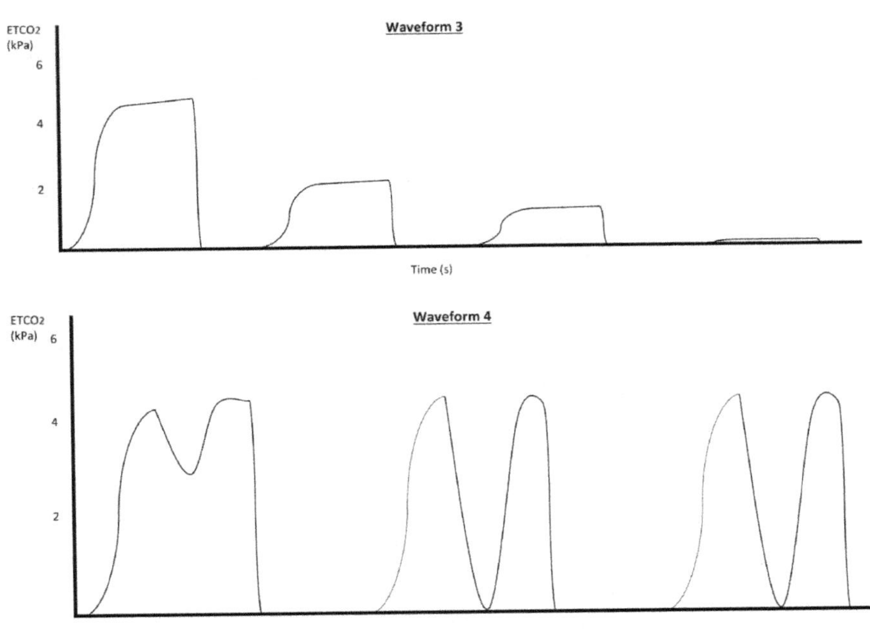
Waveform 3
ETCO2 (kPa)
6
4
2
Time (s)
Waveform 4
ETCO2 (kPa)
6
4
2
Time (s)

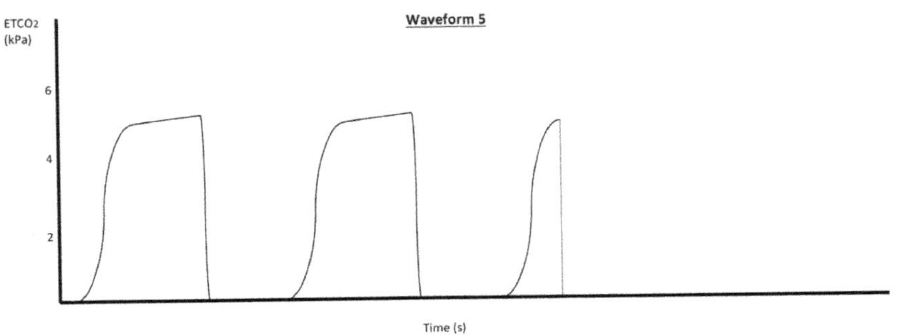
Waveform 5
ETCO2 (kPa)
6
4
2
Time (s)

**DATA INTERPRETATION OSCE – WAVEFORM CAPNOGRAPHY ANALYSIS**

| Task | Achieved | Not Achieved |
|---|---|---|
| Introduces self. | | |
| Establishes student ODP's baseline knowledge. | | |
| Explains that capnography demonstrates how CO2 partial pressure changes over the respiratory cycle. Demonstrates inspiration and expiration on graph. | | |
| Used to confirm correct placement of endo-tracheal tube. | | |
| Used to demonstrate the adequacy of ventilation | | |
| Used in cardiac arrest to assess adequacy of cardiopulmonary resuscitation or return of spontaneous circulation. | | |
| Waveform One – identifies normal waveform. | | |
| Waveform Two – identifies obstructive waveform. | | |
| Waveform Two – suggests causes include equipment problems e.g. kinking or blockage of ETT/Airway Device and pathological causes e.g. COPD, bronchospasm, laryngospasm. | | |
| Waveform Two – actions include checking patency of airway device and circuit, and examining patient for signs of upper and lower airway obstruction. | | |
| Waveform Three – identifies sudden loss of cardiac output | | |
| Waveform Three – suggests cause is cardiac arrest, or massive PE. | | |
| Waveform Three – actions include looking for signs of life, instituting resuscitation, identifying and correcting reversible causes. | | |
| Waveform Four – identifies spontaneous respiratory effort against ventilator. | | |
| Waveform Four – causes include insufficient neuromuscular blockade, increased painful stimuli, insufficient depth of anaesthesia. | | |
| Waveform Four – actions include administering further neuromuscular blockade/analgesia/anaesthetic, or assessing if appropriate to allow spontaneous breathing. | | |
| Waveform Five – identifies likely disconnection in breathing circuit or capnography line. | | |
| Waveform Five – check that airway device still in-situ, look for and correct disconnection in circuit or monitoring. | | |
| Presents information in structured manner. | | |
| Checks student's understanding, allows opportunity for questions. | | |
| Examiner's global mark | /5 | |
| Actor's global mark | /5 | |
| Total station mark | /30 | |

## Learning Points

- End-tidal CO2 monitoring, or Capnography, is essential to anaesthetic practice; it confirms correct placement of an endotracheal tube, and allows us to assess the adequacy of ventilation.

- End-tidal CO2 monitoring also gives information about the adequacy of cardiac output, and can detect low output states or sudden events such as a PE or Cardiac Arrest.

- Abnormalities in the capnography trace can arise from a clinical problem, e.g. COPD or bronchospasm, or from an equipment issue i.e. kinking of the endotracheal tube. A systematic review of both patient and breathing circuit is required to identify and correct the problem.

# DATA INTERPRETATION OSCE - Arterial blood gas analysis

## Candidate's Instructions:

Richard, patient ID 1234567D, is a 36-year-old man with a history of heroin and crack cocaine use who has presented to the Emergency Department with difficulty breathing and a productive cough. He has been triaged and 60% oxygen is being administered via a Venturi mask.

You are a Foundation Year 1 doctor working in the Emergency Department and you have been asked to review his arterial blood gas. This is shown below;

| ID: 1234567D, Richard, arterial, 01/01/2016, 10:20am | | |
|---|---|---|
| pH | 7.30 | |
| $pO_2$ | 10.1 | kPa |
| $pCO_2$ | 3.5 | kPa |
| $HCO_3$ | 20 | mmol/L |
| Lactate | 3.5 | mmol/L |
| BE | -5 | |
| Na+ | 137 | mmol/L |
| Cl- | 101 | mmol/L |
| Hb | 157 | g/L |

Review the information and when then summarise your findings and plan of action to the ED registrar.

## Examiner's Instructions:

Richard is a 28-year-old man who has presented to the ED acutely short of breath and with a productive cough.

He has a history of heroin and crack cocaine use.

As part of his work up today he has had an arterial blood gas taken.

The candidate should interpret the results and summarise their findings. The SpR will then ask them the following questions.

- What they would like to do next?
- What tests they would like (if any)?
- What their treatment would be if the CXR showed consolidation of the Right Middle Lobe?
- What changes may they see on the arterial blood gas if the patient was tiring?
- How they would treat the lactic acidosis?
- What arterial PO2 they would expect with an inspired oxygen concentration of 60% in a healthy subject?

## Actor's Instructions:

You are a Registrar covering the Emergency Department. You have performed an arterial blood gas on Richard, a 28 year old male who has presented to hospital acutely short of breath. He is currently having 60% oxygen via venturi mask.

The Foundation year 1 Doctor has been asked to to interpret the blood gas and present their findings to you.

When they have finished, you should ask them the following questions:

- What they would like to do next?
- What tests they would like (if any)?
- What their treatment would be if the CXR showed consolidation of the Right Middle Lobe?
- What changes may they see on the arterial blood gas if the patient was tiring?
- How they would treat the lactic acidosis?
- What arterial PO2 they would expect with an inspired oxygen concentration of 60% in a healthy subject?

**DATA INTERPRETATION OSCE - Arterial blood gas analysis**

| Task: | Achieved | Not Achieved |
|---|---|---|
| Verifies this is a arterial blood gas from the correct patient at the correct time | | |
| Identifies acidaemia | | |
| Identifies hypoxia | | |
| Identifies hypocapnia | | |
| Identifies a metabolic/lactic acidosis | | |
| Identifies normal sodium and chloride level | | |
| Identifies mildly elevated haemoglobin level | | |
| Identifies raised A-a gradient | | |
| Identifies Type 1 respiratory failure | | |
| Identifies concurrent metabolic acidosis with partial respiratory compensation | | |
| Gives sensible differential diagnoses (e.g. infection, bronchospasm, PE, pneumothorax) | | |
| States they would take a history and examine the patient | | |
| States they would obtain baseline physiological observations | | |
| States they would titrate oxygen to obtain a $SpO_2$ of ≥94% | | |
| Would order tests directed towards their differential diagnoses (Accept any 2 of: CXR, CT-PA, urinary pneumococcal antigen, atypical screen, HIV test, baseline biochemistry, sputum and blood cultures) | | |
| Recognises that the patient is unwell and asks for senior help | | |
| Treats consolidation with antibiotics and can name an appropriate antibiotic regimen e.g. co-amoxiclav and clarithromycin.<br>Stating 'I would check the hospital guidelines for community acquired pneumonia is acceptable'. | | |
| States that the $pCO_2$ would rise and the pH would fall if the patient was tiring | | |
| States that lactic acidosis is treated with a fluid bolus | | |
| States expected PO2 50kPa (accept 45-52 kPa) | | |
| Examiner's Global Mark | /5 | |
| Actor / Helper's Global Mark | /5 | |
| Total station mark | /30 | |

## Learning Points

Although blood gas analysis is important, it should never supplant taking a history and performing a thorough examination.

Have a systematic approach to interpretation of blood gases

Is the pH normal?
Is the $pO_2$ adequate?
Determine the respiratory component ($pCO_2$)
Determine the metabolic component ($HCO_3$, Base excess)

- In a young, otherwise healthy individual, a normal $pO_2$ on air is 13.6 kPa. A low $pO_2$ (e.g. the 10kPa seen in this case) despite supplementary oxygen is concerning and indicates a raised alveolar-arterial (A-a) gradient, the commonest cause of which is V:Q mismatch. As a simple rule of thumb, the arterial pO2 should be about 10 less than the inspired oxygen concentration. This difference is physiological and represents the addition of water vapour (humidification) and mixing with alveolar CO2.

# DATA INTERPRETATION OSCE – ABG ANALYSIS II

## Candidate's instructions:

You are the Foundation Year 1 working in the Intensive Care Unit. One of the critical care nurses requests your assistance interpreting an Arterial Blood Gas she has performed on Kalyani, a 73-year old admitted with an infective exacerbation of COPD. The nurse is concerned that the patient has become more drowsy over the past 4 hours.

You must initially talk through your interpretation of the ABG to the new nurse and outline a brief plan. After six minutes summarise your findings and the likely diagnosis to the examiner and answer some questions they will ask you.

## Results

Arterial blood gas: 23/09/16 18:45
Kalyani, DOB 7/5/1943
fiO2 0.3

| | |
|---|---|
| pH | 7.23 |
| $P_aO_2$ | 7.2kPa |
| $P_aCO_2$ | 8.8kPa |
| $HCO_3^-$ | 36mmol/L |
| Base excess | 4mmol/L |

## Examiner's instructions

Kalyani is a 73-year old admitted with an infective exacerbation of COPD. The Critical Care Outreach nurse is concerned that the patient has become more drowsy over the past 4 hours. Please ask the candidate to review the ABG which has been performed, present the findings and suggest the likely diagnosis.

Please complete the station by asking the following questions:

- What would you do next?
- What further investigations would you request for this patient?
- What management would you institute?
- What other causes of a respiratory acidosis do you know?

## Results

Arterial blood gas: 23/09/16 18:45
Kalyani, DOB 7/5/1943
fiO2 0.3

| | |
|---|---|
| pH | 7.23 |
| $P_aO_2$ | 7.2kPa |
| $P_aCO_2$ | 8.8kPa |
| $HCO_3^-$ | 36mmol/L |
| Base excess | 4mmol/L |

## Actor's instructions

Kalyani is a 73-year old admitted with an infective exacerbation of COPD. You are the new Critical Care nurse looking after the patient and are concerned that she has become more drowsy over the past 4 hours. You have returned to work after a 5 year career break and although you are previously trained at looking at blood gases you currently don't feel hugely confident with them so have asked the doctor on the ward for some help with interpreting the ABG.

Please ask the candidate to review the ABG which has been performed, present the findings and suggest the likely diagnosis. They will then need to summarise their findings to the examiner and answer some direct Qs.

## Results

Arterial blood gas: 23/09/16 18:45
Kalyani, DOB 7/5/1943
fiO2 0.3

| | |
|---|---|
| pH | 7.23 |
| $P_aO_2$ | 7.2kPa |
| $P_aCO_2$ | 8.8kPa |
| $HCO_3^-$ | 36mmol/L |
| Base excess | 4mmol/L |

**DATA INTERPRETATION OSCE – ABG ANALYSIS**

| Task | Achieved | Not Achieved |
|---|---|---|
| Introduces self | | |
| Checks Nurse's name and role and clarifies clinical situation and concern | | |
| Confirms patient details | | |
| Confirms date and time of sample | | |
| Comments on the pH and level of acidity | | |
| Comments on oxygenation | | |
| Determines any respiratory component | | |
| Determines any metabolic component | | |
| Outlines primary disturbance –type 2 respiratory failure with respiratory acidosis | | |
| States the presence of partial metabolic compensation | | |
| Suggests diagnosis – respiratory failure due to exacerbation of COPD | | |
| Mentions A-E approach in initial assessment of patient | | |
| Suggests initial management plan – nebulized salbutamol and ipratropium, steroids, antibiotics if evidence of infection. | | |
| Understands need for controlled O2 therapy | | |
| Suggests need for Non-Invasive Ventilation | | |
| Mentions other investigations – CXR, Blood tests including CRP, FBC, Blood cultures, Atypical Pneumonia Screen. (Accept any 3) | | |
| Mentions would request senior support | | |
| Outlines importance of regular clinical assessment and repeated ABGs to assess response to treatment | | |
| States other causes of respiratory acidosis e.g. head injury, opioid over-dose, constrictive chest wall deformities, chest trauma(Accept any 2) | | |
| Summarises data to examiner in structured manner | | |
| | | |
| Examiner's global mark | /5 | |
| Actor's global mark | /5 | |
| Total station mark | /30 | |

## Learning Points

- An ABG should always be assessed in combination with a clinical review of the patient. We treat patients, not numbers!

- Patients with chronic respiratory disease may chronically retain CO2, leading to a compensatory high bicarbonate level on the ABG.

- Patients with COPD and Type 2 Respiratory Failure who have a pH < 7.26 should be considered for a trial of Non-Invasive Ventilation. These patients must be reviewed regularly and may be best suited to an HDU environment where insertion of an arterial line allows for regular ABG sampling. Those who fail to improve may need intubation and invasive ventilation, though this will not be suitable for every patient and senior decision making is mandatory.

# DATA INTERPRETATION OSCE – ABG ANALYSIS III

## Candidate's instructions:

A 22-year-old man, Tom, has been brought in to the emergency department after having been found drowsy and unwell at home by his friend. She says he has been ill for a few days with severe vomiting and abdominal pain.

You are the Foundation year doctor in the department and have been asked by a senior colleague to analyse and comment on the following arterial blood gas result from the patient, to aid management of his condition.

After evaluating the blood gas you should present it to the examiner and answer any questions they may have.

## Results

Arterial blood gas: 3/8/16 16:45
Mr Tom, DOB 15/5/95
fiO2 0.21

| | |
|---|---|
| pH | 6.94 |
| $P_aO_2$ | 13.8kPa |
| $P_aCO_2$ | 2.5kPa |
| $HCO_3^-$ | 8mmol/L |
| Base excess | -19.5mmol/L |
| Glucose | 27mmol/L |

## Examiner's instructions

A 22-year-old man is brought to the emergency department semi conscious with a prior history of severe vomiting and abdominal pain.

The patient is being resuscitated and assessed by an ED doctor, who has asked the F1 doctor to analyse and interpret an arterial blood gas sample in order to manage the patient.

Allow 6 minutes for the candidate to present the data in a structured manner, and then summarise their analysis. When they have presented their findings, ask the following questions:

- What is the likely diagnosis?
- What further investigations would you order in this patient?
- What management would you institute?
- What other causes of a metabolic acidosis do you know?

## Results

Arterial blood gas: 3/8/16 16:45
Mr Tom, DOB 15/5/95
fiO2 0.21

| | |
|---|---|
| pH | 6.94 |
| $P_aO_2$ | 13.8kPa |
| $P_aCO_2$ | 2.5kPa |
| $HCO_3^-$ | 8mmol/L |
| Base excess | -19.5mmol/L |
| Glucose | 27mmol/L |

**DATA INTERPRETATION OSCE – ABG ANALYSIS**

| Task | Achieved | Not Achieved |
|---|---|---|
| Introduces self | | |
| Confirms patient details | | |
| Confirms date and time of sample | | |
| Comments on the pH and level of acidity | | |
| Comments on oxygenation | | |
| Determines any respiratory component | | |
| Determines the metabolic component | | |
| Comments on hyperglycaemia | | |
| Outlines primary disturbance – severe metabolic acidosis | | |
| States the presence of partial respiratory compensation | | |
| Suggests diagnosis – Diabetic ketoacidosis | | |
| Mentions other investigations – blood or urinary ketones, tests for possible precipitating cause | | |
| Mentions A-E approach in initial resuscitation of patient | | |
| Suggests initial management plan – fluid replacement and insulin, | | |
| Outlines importance of regular blood glucose and pH monitoring | | |
| Discusses potassium replacement | | |
| Suggests definitive management – diabetes control, treatment of any underlying conditions | | |
| States other causes of metabolic acidosis | | |
| Presents data in structured manner | | |
| Sensible approach to management of DKA | | |
| | | |
| Examiner's global mark | /5 | |
| Actor's global mark | /5 | |
| Total station mark | /30 | |

## Learning Points

- Having a clear structure when analysing data is important in helping process relevant information, especially in high-pressure situations. However obvious the abnormalities on a piece of data may seem, always stick to your chosen system to ensure you don't miss other concurrent issues.

- Arterial blood gases are invaluable in providing essential information about patient physiology in emergency circumstances as well as useful monitoring tools. Becoming familiar with interpreting them will greatly improve clinical practice.

- Metabolic acidosis is usually a medical emergency. The A-E approach in managing patients is critical but also be aware of the common causes and treatments.

# CRITICAL CARE OSCE – Bleeding oesophageal varices

## Candidate's Instructions:

You are the Foundation Year 1 covering the Acute Medical Unit. You are asked to see Samuel, a 53-year-old patient whose GP has referred him for investigation of ascites. The nurse admitting him is concerned that his blood pressure is low.

After 6 minutes the examiner will stop you and ask you to summarise back your findings, suggest your management plan and answer some direct questions.

## Examiner's Instructions:

Samuel is a 53-year-old patient with alcohol dependence whose GP has referred him for investigation of ascites. The nurse admitting him is concerned that his blood pressure is low.

The admitting nurse has noticed that he has a tachycardia of 120 and blood pressure of 75/40.

The candidate should perform an ABCDE assessment which will reveal signs of hypovolaemia and presence of malaena.

They should concurrently take a basic history which should reveal the patient's excessive alcohol consumption, and a 2-day history of copious amounts of black offensive stools.

The patient will deteriorate during the station with signs of worsening haemorrhagic shock. The candidate will be expected to administer fluids and request flying squad/O -ve blood in addition to calling for appropriate help.

In the final two minutes, ask them to provide a differential diagnosis, outline what abnormalities they will be looking for in laboratory investigations, and state that the patient will require an urgent OGD. Establish if they understand the rationale for antibiotic therapy and terlipressin.

## Assistant's Instructions:

You are an experienced staff nurse who has asked the candidate to see Samuel, a 53-year-old man whose GP has referred him for investigation of ascites.

You are concerned that your admission observations reveal of heart rate of 120 and blood pressure of 75/40.

Direct the candidate to make an assessment of the mannequin. Initial findings will be as follows;

**A**: Talking in full sentences, but complaining of feeling light headed and nauseated.
**B**: RR 26, SpO2 96% on air, otherwise normal.
**C**: Cold, clammy peripheries up to shoulders. Central capillary refill less than 4 seconds. Regular radial pulse rate of 120/min, blood pressure 75/40.
**D**: Responds to voice/GCS 14 (eye opens to voice.) Pupils 3mm, equal and reactive, BM 5.
**E**: Temperature 36. Spider Naevi over chest wall. Distended abdomen (ascites). Malaena on bed sheets.

As the station progresses, the patient will continue to bleed and their condition will deteriorate with falling conscious level and worsening haemodynamic instability.

If the candidate asks for further history, the patient takes no regular medications, but has drank excessive alcohol for over 10 years. He currently drinking 1L of vodka and 10 cans of super-strength lager per day. His GP referred him to the medical team this morning for investigation of ascites. If questioned about bowel habit, the patient will report 2 days of large amounts of offensive, black, runny stool.
**You are an experienced nurse who is able to assist the candidate in initiating any treatment which they feel is appropriate.**

**CRITICAL CARE OSCE – Bleeding oesophageal varices**

| Task: | Achieved | Not Achieved |
|---|---|---|
| Introduces self to patient and seeks permission to perform assessment | | |
| Takes focused history of acute problem – offensive black stools, asks about haematemesis | | |
| Brief past medical and drug history including allergy status | | |
| Social history, identifies excessive alcohol consumption | | |
| Performs A to E assessment | | |
| Picks up on clinical signs of hypovolaemia | | |
| Recognises Upper GI Bleed as cause | | |
| Calls for appropriate help – e.g. 2222/Major Haemorrhage call, senior doctor, ICU | | |
| Gives 10-15L of Oxygen using non-rebreathe mask | | |
| Establishes IV access, recognizes need for multiple sites/wide bore access | | |
| Sends relevant blood tests including Crossmatch sample, FBC, Coag/INR, U&Es, LFTs | | |
| Gives IV fluid bolus | | |
| Gives O-negative blood | | |
| Repeats A to E assessment following fluid/blood transfusion | | |
| Requests other blood products – FFP, Platelets | | |
| Requests IV Antibiotics and knows rationale for this | | |
| Requests terlipressin and knows rationale for this | | |
| Aware of need for urgent OGD | | |
| Summarises case to examiner | | |
| Remains calm and methodical throughout | | |
| | | |
| Examiner's Global Mark | /5 | |
| Actor / Helper's Global Mark | /5 | |
| Total Station Mark | /30 | |

## Learning Points

- Oesophageal varices are dilated veins, vulnerable to bleeding, which occur in patients with portal hypertension. They can be a cause of major haemorrhage.

- An OGD is required to identify and treat the bleeding, which may include banding or sclerotherapy. As a last resort compression of the varices with a Sengstaken-Blakemore tube may be required but this will only be performed by senior doctors in parallel with intubation.

- NICE Guidelines recommend giving terlipressin and IV Antibiotics in the acute treatment of variceal Bleeding. The former aims to reduce portal hypertension and reduce the pressure in the varices, while the latter reduces the incidence of hepatic-encephalopathy.

# CRITICAL CARE OSCE – UNCONSCIOUS PATIENT

## Candidate's instructions.

A 72-year-old man was admitted under the medical take earlier in the day for treatment of pneumonia, but has now been found unconscious by a staff nurse.

You are the Foundation Year 1 doctor on call and have been asked to assess and treat the patient appropriately.

After 6 minutes the examiner will stop you and ask you to summarise back your findings and suggest your management plan.

## Examiner's instructions

A 72-year-old man, admitted to a medical ward for treatment of pneumonia, is found unconscious by a staff nurse.

The Foundation Year 1 doctor has been asked to assess and treat the patient appropriately. The candidate is to use an A-E approach and may ask for relevant history and investigations, results of which would be provided.

Stop the candidates after 6 minutes and ask them to summarise the case. Then ask them:

- what other medications would you prescribe on the drug chart to be used in the event of recurrent hypoglycaemia?
- what is the target capillary blood glucose level for a patient with critical illness?

## Actor's instructions

You are a staff nurse working on the medical ward. You have called the Foundation Year 1 doctor to see a patient who you found unconscious in bed.

He is a 72-year-old man being treated for pneumonia. He also has a history of hypertension and Type 2 Diabetes. He has eaten little today due to nausea but has received his regular medications (Amlodipine and Insulin). He has no allergies and no relatives available for a collateral history.

You will assist the doctor with any requests and provide appropriate results.

## Results

Observations

Respiratory rate - 24
Heart rate – 116bpm
Blood pressure – 96/64mmHg
Temperature – 37.9°C
Oxygen saturation – 91% on room air

Examination findings

A - Airway patent with no abnormal sounds

B - Equal chest expansion bilaterally
- Trachea central
- Dull percussion note in right base
- Bronchial breathing in right lower zone

C - Cool, clammy patient with generalised pallor
- Palpable central and peripheral pulses – regular rhythm with tachycardia
- Normal heart sounds

D - AVPU on alertness scale; GCS – 6/15 (E1V1M4)
- Capillary blood glucose – 2.3mmol/L
- Dilated pupils, equal and reactive

E - No signs of trauma or injury
- Normal abdominal examination
- No focal neurological deficit

**COMMUNICATION OSCE – UNCONSCIOUS PATIENT**

| Task | Achieved | Not Achieved |
|---|---|---|
| Ensures safe to approach, wears gloves | | |
| Confirms patient identity and asks for background information | | |
| Requests appropriate help (e.g. periarrest team/Medical Emergency Team call) | | |
| Checks for signs of life - rules out cardiac arrest | | |
| Checks physiological observations/attaches monitoring | | |
| Airway assessment – confirms airway patency by looking, listening and feeling | | |
| Breathing assessment – including application of high flow oxygen | | |
| Circulation assessment – including intravenous access and blood tests | | |
| Disability assessment – checks consciousness level and blood glucose | | |
| Immediately treats hypoglycaemia using intravenous Dextrose (e.g. 100ml 20% dextrose then reassesses patient) | | |
| Exposure - looking for rashes, injuries etc | | |
| States will continually reassess conscious level and recheck capillary glucose after treatment | | |
| Reviews patient notes and charts for further history – states medications to be reviewed | | |
| Discusses with appropriate seniors – states will consider ITU if remains unconscious | | |
| Identifies oral glucose gel & IM glucagon as additional treatments of hypoglycaemia | | |
| States capillary glucose range of 6-10mmol/l for critically ill patients | | |
| Gives concise and accurate summary | | |
| Suggests definitive management for hypoglycaemia including regular blood sugar monitoring | | |
| Systematic assessment of patient | | |
| Professional approach to managing patient | | |
| Examiner's global mark | /5 | |
| Actor's global mark | /5 | |
| Total station mark | /30 | |

## Learning Points

- The causes of a depressed conscious level are numerous - a structured A-E approach is essential to ensure that no reversible causes are missed! Remember 'DEFG' stands for 'Don't Ever Forget Glucose'!

- Identification and immediate correction of abnormal physiology is a core part of the A-E assessment. Early reassessment after initiating an intervention is essential in both the OSCE and real life clinical scenarios.

- Abnormalities of plasma blood glucose levels commonly accompany critical illness. The 'stress response' is associated with insulin resistance and hyperglycaemia, but the patient may also become hypoglycaemic if they receive hypoglycaemic agents when they are not eating properly. A variable rate intravenous insulin infusion ('sliding-scale') will ensure that the patient has their blood sugar checked regularly and that their insulin doses match their requirements.

# CRITICAL CARE OSCE – Amitriptyline Overdose

## Candidate's Instructions:

You are a Foundation Year 1 doing your Emergency Department rotation. You are asked to urgently assess Lena, a 19-year-old woman brought to resus by ambulance. She is unconscious and hypotensive. Her mother called the ambulance having found her collapsed in her bedroom – she has been worried about her mood and behavior since Lena failed her first-year university exams.

You have been asked to assess and stabilise the patient and start initial management.

After 6 minutes the examiner will stop you and ask you to summarise back your findings and suggest your management plan from here on.

## Examiner's Instructions:

Lena is a 19-year-old woman who has been brought to the Emergency Department by ambulance. She was found unconscious by her mother, who has been concerned about Lena's low mood and erratic behaviour since she failed her first-year exams.

The candidate should perform an A to E assessment, where they will discover signs of tricyclic overdose.

If they probe for further history, the paramedic is able to report that Lena's mother takes Amitriptyline for back pain, and several empty packets of the drug were found hidden in a bin in the bathroom.

The candidate should begin appropriate resuscitation while requesting senior help and support from ICU/Anaesthetics. In the final two minutes ask them to summarise the case and list the clinical features of Tricyclic overdose. If not clear from the scenario, clarify whether they know how to obtain information on treating a potential poisoning or drug overdose, and if they know of a specific intervention for tricyclic poisoning.

## Assistant's Instructions:

You are the paramedic who brought Lena, a 19-year-old woman to the Emergency Department resus. Her mother called for an ambulance having discovered her daughter unconscious at home.

Direct the candidate to perform an examination of the mannequin and treat any problems they identify.

If they seek evidence of poisoning or overdose, hand them empty packets of amitriptyline, which Lena's mother takes for back pain. State that the mother is concerned her daughter may have self-harmed, as Lena has been low in mood since failing her university exams.

An ABCDE examination will reveal:

**A**: Snoring, which improves with simple airway manoeuvres and an airway adjunct
**B**: RR 10, SpO2 96% on air, otherwise normal
**C**: Warm peripheries, radial pulse normal volume, regular at 120 beats per minute, BP 90/50, CRT 2 seconds.
**D**: Responds to pain, GCS 7 E1V2M4. Pupils 6mm, equal and reactive. BM 5.
**E**: Temperature 37. Nil of note.

Following the initial assessment, the candidate may ask you to perform certain tasks or administer medications.

We would expect them to request;

Senior Help – in particular they may state they need an anesthetist to manage the airway. Tell them you have bleeped for assistance, but there may be a delay in help arriving.
Oxygen – 15L via a Non Re-Breathe Mask.
Airway Adjuncts – they may request either oropharyngeal or nasaopharyngeal airways; offer a selection of sizes so they can

demonstrate correct sizing. Offer to take over the maintenance of airway manoeuvers, e.g. jaw thrust.

IV Access – they may also request blood tests, including Paracetamol/Salicylate levels.

Arterial Blood Gas - after a delay for processing show them results with pH 7.22, PaCO2 6.8 kPA, PaO2 25 kPA, HCO3 20, BE -3.5, Lac 3.0

ECG – produce a 12 lead ECG showing a prolonged QRS interval; ask the candidate to explain the findings to you.

Drugs and IV Fluids – in particular they may request Sodium Bicarbonate.

National Poisoning Information Service – they may ask you to consult "Toxbase" for information on amitriptyline overdose, tell them the nurse-in-charge is looking for this.

**CRITICAL CARE OSCE – Amitriptyline Overdose**

| Task: | Achieved | Not Achieved |
|---|---|---|
| Introduces self to patient/assistant and seeks permission to perform assessment | | |
| Seeks further history, recognizes potential for amitriptyline overdose | | |
| Performs A to E assessment | | |
| Recognises partial airway obstruction | | |
| Correctly performs simple airway manoeuvres | | |
| Correctly sizes and inserts an oropharyngeal or nasopharyngeal airway | | |
| Requests assistance i.e. anaesthetics/ICU to manage airway | | |
| Gives 10-15L of Oxygen using non-rebreathe mask | | |
| Establishes IV access | | |
| Requests appropriate blood tests including paracetamol/salicylate levels | | |
| Administers IV Fluids | | |
| Requests and correctly interprets ABG | | |
| Requests and correctly interprets 12 Lead ECG | | |
| Seeks further information regarding tricyclic poisoning from poisons advice service (eg NPIS/Toxbase) | | |
| Requests Sodium Bicarbonate infusion, or aware that this may be appropriate | | |
| States need for ICU admission | | |
| Reassesses after interventions | | |
| Summarises case to examiner | | |
| Can describe the signs and symptoms associated with tricyclic overdose | | |
| Remains calm and methodical throughout | | |
| | | |
| Examiner's Global Mark | /5 | |
| Actor / Helper's Global Mark | /5 | |
| Total Station Mark | /30 | |

## Learning Points

• Tricyclic antidepressants such as Amitriptyline are dangerous in overdose. Their anticholinergic effects lead to tachycardia, pupillary dilatation, urinary retention, dry mouth and sedation; sodium and calcium channel blockade causes myocardial toxicity, with conduction delays producing broad QRS complexes and ventricular arrhythmias; alpha-receptor blockade causes hypotension.

• Management of tricyclic overdose is largely supportive, but the administration of Sodium Bicarbonate can be useful, as it reverses the metabolic acidosis. A more alkaline pH increases the amount of amitriptyline bound to plasma proteins and hence reduces the amount of free drug available to exert its effects. It may also reverse the direct myocardial effects.

• In any suspected poisoning, the National Poisons Information Service can provide useful information via their Toxbase website or telephone line. Toxicology is rarely a service that hospitals have on site so it is essential to utilise their online resources and print out the recommendations to remain in the patient notes.

# CRITICAL CARE OSCE – Status Epilepticus

## Candidate's Instructions:

You are a Foundation Year 1 on your anaesthetics placement. You are on the medical ward to pre-assess a patient for surgery on behalf of your consultant (who is in theatre). As you enter the bay the nursing staff call you over to a different patient who is having seizures.

Jonny is a 24-year-old patient with a history of epilepsy who is undergoing treatment with IV antibiotics for a community acquired pneumonia. His seizures are usually well controlled with oral sodium valproate.

After 6 minutes the examiner will stop you and ask you to summarise back your findings, suggest your management plan and ask you some direct questions.

## Examiner's Instructions:

Jonny is a 24-year-old patient with a history of epilepsy (generalised seizures). His epilepsy is normally well controlled with twice daily oral sodium valproate (300mg). He has been an in-patient on the medical ward since yesterday, requiring treatment with IV antibiotics for community-acquired pneumonia. He is penicillin allergic, so is being treated with IV levofloxacin.

The patient has been having generalised seizures on the ward for 7 minutes now, and has not responded to initial buccal midazolam by the nursing staff. He has jaw clenching, but with high flow oxygen through a reservoir mask has maintained saturations of 96%. He is tachycardic (105 beats per minute), has normal blood pressure (134/69), and is apyrexial (temperature 37.4).

The candidate has been asked to assist in the immediate management by nursing staff, and should assess the patient with an ABCDE approach. The scenario requires knowledge of the step-wise approach to the management of status epilepticus.

With 2 minutes remaining ask the candidate for possible causes of the onset of seizures – relevant to this scenario these would include acute infection and pharmacological interaction (with a quinolone antibiotic). If it has not been volunteered enquire about escalation of care for refractory status epilepticus.

## Actor's Instructions:

You are a senior staff nurse in charge of the bay on a medical ward. You have been looking after Jonny during your last two shifts. He is receiving 500mg levofloxacin IV twice daily to treat his pneumonia (he is penicillin allergic) and has been doing well. As far as you know he had been seizure-free for over a year, and was administered his normal doses of sodium valproate on the ward last night and this morning. His seizure started abruptly 7 minutes ago, with generalised tonic-clonic pattern when he was lying in bed. He hasn't bitten his tongue, but does have a clenched jaw and an erratic breathing pattern.

You have alerted the patient's own medical team, but haven't initiated a priority call. After 5 minutes of seizures you administered a single dose of buccal midazolam (10mg) and applied oxygen through a reservoir mask, but have given no intravenous medications, as they are not prescribed. The patient is still on his back, and you haven't managed to move the patient into a lateral position yet.

His cannula is patent and working well. You would like to know what to do next, in particular which medications should be prescribed and given. You think this is status epilepticus and are worried about what to do if the seizures do not terminate with initial treatment.

**CRITICAL CARE OSCE – Status epilepticus**

| Task: | Achieved | Not Achieved |
|---|---|---|
| Identifies self to team | | |
| Mentions initial assessment of ABCDE | | |
| States would attempt airway manoeuvres (head-tilt, chin-lift) | | |
| Requests airway adjunct (e.g., nasopharyngeal airway) | | |
| Requests suction | | |
| Ensures high flow oxygen administration | | |
| Mentions measurement of blood glucose | | |
| Ensures adequate intravenous access | | |
| Clarifies timing of onset of seizures | | |
| Clarifies customary anti-epileptic drugs and treatment initiated so far | | |
| Checks allergy status | | |
| Requests administration of IV lorazepam | | |
| Offers dosage of IV lorazepam (0.1mg/kg, up to 4mg) | | |
| Requests intravenous loading dose of phenytoin (dosage of phenytoin not required to be known (15 – 18 mg/kg) | | |
| Declares diagnosis of status epilepticus | | |
| Able to name subsequent pharmacological agents for persistent seizures (phenobarbitaone, thiopentone) | | |
| Calls for senior help / medical emergency team | | |
| Summarises finding back to examiner | | |
| Indicates potential need for escalation - general anaesthetic / intensive care | | |
| Able to identify potential causes for seizure onset (e.g., infection, antibiotic interaction) | | |
| | | |
| Examiner's Global Mark | /5 | |
| Actor / Helper's Global Mark | /5 | |
| Total Station Mark | /30 | |

## Learning Points

- Patients with epilepsy frequently present to hospital with acute illnesses, often unrelated to their disease. Common triggers for seizures include missed anti-epileptic drug doses, poor compliance with medication, alcohol use, infection, and drug interactions. It is particularly important to check for interactions when prescribing acutely as certain medications can reduce seizure threshold (in this case, a quinolone).

- The definition of status epilepticus traditionally required seizures to persist for longer than 20-30 minutes or for patients to have further seizures without returning to full consciousness in between fits. This is now evolving to recognise that most seizure episodes will terminate spontaneously within 2 – 3 minutes. Therefore, generalised tonic-clonic seizures lasting beyond 5 minutes may represent status epilepticus and require early proactive treatment.

- The majority of hospitals will adhere to advanced life support seizure algorithms, however As epilepsy pharmacotherapy advances, newer agents (for example, levetiracetam) are likely to be incorporated into these treatment algorithms in place of older drugs (that are associated with significant side effects). It is important to remain up to date with current specialist guidance. Known epileptics may also have bespoke management plans in place.

# CRITICAL CARE OSCE – Septic shock

## Candidate's Instructions:

You are a Foundation Year 1 on your ICU placement. You are attending a patient in the Emergency Department ahead of your registrar who is due to join you imminently.

Tim is a 78-year-old gentleman with a history of benign prostatic hypertrophy, who has been moved to the Resus area after becoming hypotensive and drowsy. He was admitted with pyrexia, vomiting and loin pain.

The charge nurse in ED looking after the patient is able to provide you with much of the salient history and is fully aware of what investigations and treatment have been initiated.

After 6 minutes the examiner will stop you and ask you to summarise back your findings, suggest your management plan and ask you some direct questions.

## Examiner's Instructions:

Tim is a 78-year-old patient with a history of benign prostatic hypertrophy who is being assessed in the Emergency Department (ED) Resus area. He has no significant past medical history, and is generally active and well, with no allergies.

For the last 18 hours he has developed left loin pain, vomiting and rigors. He had a temperature of 38.9°C on arrival to the ED 20 minutes ago and was normotensive with a tachycardia of 108 beats/minute. He now has a blood pressure of 85/37mmHg, and tachycardia at a rate of 113/min. He is drowsy and much less responsive than when he arrived.

The ED staff have inserted a large bore IV cannula, and are administering a bolus of 250ml crystalloid. They sent routine bloods (FBC, UE, CRP), but no serum lactate measurement or blood cultures when the cannula was inserted. He has received no antibiotics.

The experienced nurse with the patient is able to provide all of the relevant history points, and can provide the candidate with details of the investigations and treatment so far.

With 2 minutes remaining the examiner should ask the candidate to present back their finding and should be asked directly to summarise the approach to treating a septic patient.

## Actor's Instructions:

You are an experienced charge nurse in the Resus area of the Emergency Department. You brought the patient Tim through from the Majors area after he dropped his blood pressure and became drowsy. He has no airway compromise, and is breathing at a rate of 26 breaths / min. He has a Glasgow Coma Score of 13 (E3, V4, M6), but is unable to give a clear history at the moment. You haven't yet managed to put an oxygen mask on him to administer oxygen.

The patient has no significant past medical history apart from an enlarged prostate. He takes no medicines and has no allergies. He has been suffering from nausea and vomiting for 18 hours, with some left loin pain. It was mildly tender on that side when the ED doctor examined him briefly. The patient has no abdominal distension or rebound tenderness, and has normal bowel sounds. He had his bowels open normally this morning.

On arrival in the ED the patient's temperature was 38.9°C with rigors. It is still elevated at 38.4C (he has been given paracetamol). He became muddled and drowsy in the main majors area, and has been moved into resus. He has a bolus of 250ml crystalloid infusing at the moment, with nothing else prescribed. He has had no antibiotics. Blood results are pending (FBC. UE, CRP), but he did not have any blood cultures or serum lactate sent when he was cannulated.

You are fully trained to perform IV cannulation, urinary catheterisation and blood tests, and administer treatment as requested. If the candidate does not initially offer a diagnosis of sepsis, enquire about their differential diagnosis. Offer to apply an oxygen mask and prepare antibiotics if a request for these is not forthcoming.

**CRITICAL CARE OSCE – Septic shock**

| Task: | Achieved | Not Achieved |
|---|---|---|
| Introduces self | | |
| Briefly clarifies presenting history | | |
| Briefly clarifies past medical history | | |
| Assesses patient using an ABCDE approach | | |
| Requests high flow oxygen administration | | |
| Requests current vital observations (PR, RR, BP, SpO2) | | |
| Requests blood glucose level | | |
| Requests serum lactate level | | |
| Requests further IV fluid bolus (up to 30ml/kg) to assess BP response | | |
| Requests urinary catheterisation and monitoring of fluid balance | | |
| Requests peripheral blood culture samples | | |
| Indicates requirement for urgent administration of broad spectrum IV antibiotics | | |
| Specifically checks patient allergy status prior to commencing IV antibiotics | | |
| Clear communication style | | |
| States would seek for senior help | | |
| Able to name 'Sepsis Six' initiative | | |
| Summarises findings and likely diagnosis back to examiner | | |
| Able to name investigations associated with Sepsis Six (lactate, BP & MAP, blood cultures) | | |
| Able to name therapies associated with Sepsis Six (fluid boluses, IV antibiotics, vasopressors) | | |
| Aware of requirement for critical care for patients with septic shock | | |
| | | |
| Examiner's Global Mark | /5 | |
| Actor / Helper's Global Mark | /5 | |
| Total Station Mark | /30 | |

## Learning Points

- Sepsis is a potentially life-threatening syndrome resulting from the body's maladaptive response to infection. Alterations in microvasculature and perfusion result in shock and can progress to multi-organ failure if not recognized and treated early. In the UK around 40 000 deaths annually are attributable to sepsis.

- In the UK the Surviving Sepsis Campaign, the UK sepsis Trust and the NICE sepsis guidelines have devised sepsis algorithms based on early warning scores. 'Care bundle' exist of the six evidence-based interventions that need to be completed in a finite time window from presentation, with the aim of preventing progression of the condition.

- Early Warning Score systems to track unwell patients help to identify those at risk of developing sepsis. These may well include a 'trigger' for in-hospital referral to critical care services to achieve appropriate higher level care, such as vasopressor drugs and invasive monitoring.

# CRITICAL CARE OSCE – Pneumothorax

## Candidate's Instructions:

You are the Foundation Year1 on call for Medicine. You are asked to review Moira, a 64-year-old patient in the Emergency Department who has presented via ambulance with shortness of breath. She has a background of COPD. Please take a brief history from the patient and perform an examination, treating any problems you identify.

After 6 minutes the examiner will stop you and ask you to summarise back your findings, suggest your management plan and ask you some direct questions.

## Examiner's Instructions:

Moira is a 64-year-old patient with a background of COPD. She has presented to the Emergency Department via ambulance with shortness of breath.

The candidate should take a history of her background and symptoms, and perform an ABCDE assessment. They should be suspicious of a right sided pneumothorax, and begin making appropriate arrangements to confirm and treat this.

The patient will then deteriorate, requiring emergency decompression of a tension pneumothorax, and the candidate should perform this (or state how they would do so.)

After six minutes ask the candidate to summarise the case and state what further definitive treatment is required in this case.

## Assistant's Instructions:

You are a staff nurse looking after Moira, a 64-year-old patient in Emergency Department who has presented via ambulance with shortness of breath. She has a background of COPD.

Direct the candidate to take a history from the mannequin and perform an examination.

Moira will give a history of COPD, diagnosed 10 years ago. She was a 30 pack year smoker, but quit successfully after her diagnosis. She takes daily inhalers and has a good exercise tolerance and quality of life. She also takes amlodipine for high blood pressure, but has no other health problems. Penicillin brings her out in a rash. She has had upper respiratory tract symptoms for the past few days, including a non-productive cough. She didn't feel short of breath until this morning, when after a prolonged bought of coughing she became very breathless.

An ABCDE examination will reveal:

**A**: Talking in full sentences, but complaining of feeling short of breath.

**B**: RR 28, SpO2 90% on air, decreased chest expansion on right side, hyper-resonant percussion note on right side, reduced air entry on right side. Trachea still central.

**C**: Warm peripheries, radial pulse good volume, regular at 90 beats per minute, BP 135/90, CRT 2 seconds.

**D**: Alert, GCS 15. Pupils 3mm, equal and reactive. BM 5.

**E**: Temperature 36.2. Calves soft, non-tender.

Following the initial assessment the candidate will be expected to administer oxygen and arrange an urgent chest x-ray. While this is being arranged, the patient will deteriorate with signs of severe respiratory distress and haemodynamic instability. On reassessment the patient will show signs of a right sided tension pneumothorax. The candidate will be expected to perform immediate needle decompression with a widebore IV cannula, after which the patient will stabilise.

**CRITICAL CARE OSCE – Pneumothorax**

| Task: | Achieved | Not Achieved |
|---|---|---|
| Introduces self to patient and seeks permission to perform assessment | | |
| Takes focused history of acute problem – sudden onset shortness of breath following coughing | | |
| Brief past medical history and establishes normal exercise tolerance | | |
| Drug history including allergy status | | |
| Social history, identifies ex-smoker | | |
| Performs ABCDE assessment | | |
| Picks up relevant clinical signs | | |
| States right sided pneumothorax likely diagnosis | | |
| Gives 10-15L of Oxygen using non-rebreathe mask | | |
| Establishes IV access | | |
| Requests CXR | | |
| Suggests chest drain likely to be needed as COPD | | |
| Recognises deterioration and repeats A to E assessment | | |
| Recognises signs of tension pneumothorax | | |
| Calls for appropriate help – e.g. 2222/Medical Registrar/Anaesthetics/ICU | | |
| Performs/Shows how to perform emergency decompression with wide bore cannula in $2^{nd}$ ICS MCL on right side | | |
| Reassesses patient following emergency decompression | | |
| Summarises case to examiner | | |
| States need for formal intercostal chest drain | | |
| Remains calm and methodical throughout | | |
| | | |
| Examiner's Global Mark | /5 | |
| Actor / Helper's Global Mark | /5 | |
| Total Station Mark | /30 | |

## Learning Points

- Patients with COPD and emphysematous disease can develop large bullae. These can rupture, leading to development of a pneumothorax. The British Thoracic (BTS) Guidelines exist to aid management of spontaneous pneumothoraces with COPD patients classified as secondary pneumothoraces.

- Tension Pneumothorax occurs when the pressure within the pleural space is so great it causes displacement of the mediastinum to the contralateral side, and compresses the heart and great vessels. This leads to a life-threatening fall in cardiac output. This is a clinical diagnosis, and treatment should not be delayed by obtaining a chest X-ray.

- The emergency treatment of a tension pneumothorax requires the insertion of a large bore cannula into the 2nd intercostal space in the mid-clavicular line on the side of the pneumothorax. This is a short term measure and close frequent clinical reassessment is needed as the tension pneumothorax can reaccumulate if the cannula becomes obstructed. An intercostal chest drain will need to be inserted to definitively treat the pneumothorax.

# CRITICAL CARE OSCE – Hyperkalaemia

## Candidate's Instructions:

You are a Foundation Year 1 doctor on your anaesthetics placement and have been asked to review a patient in the acute medical unit by your consultant. The staff have asked for assistance in cannulation, as the patient is dehydrated.

Heather is a 72-year-old woman with a history of hypertension, ischaemic heart disease, and chronic kidney disease (stage 3). She has been referred in by her GP as she has had very little oral intake for 2 days whilst suffering from a migraine, and has been having dizzy spells.

After 6 minutes the examiner will stop you and ask you to summarise your findings, suggest your management plan and ask you some direct questions.

## Examiner's Instructions:

Heather is a 72-year-old patient with a history of hypertension, ischaemic heart disease, chronic kidney disease and headaches. She has been admitted to the acute medical unit via her GP after becoming dehydrated with poor oral intake associated with a migraine. She is currently feeling very faint, and has become vague in her responses.

She is treated with bisoprolol, lisinopril, amlodipine regularly, with sumitriptan as required for migraine. She has no allergies. She has been taking her regular medicines, alongside paracetamol and ibuprofen for this particularly bad bout of migraine. She has been nauseated, and has had minimal oral intake.

In this scenario the combination of comorbidities, poor fluid intake, and recent medication use has led to an acute worsening of her kidney function. Her GP has referred her to the acute medical unit after performing baseline blood tests (full blood count, urea and electrolytes, C-reactive protein). These are available and reveal hyperkalaemia (6.9 mmol/L), and impaired renal function. The candidate is required to recognise this as a medical emergency and treat the hyperkalaemia accordingly.

The candidate will be prompted by the nurse in the scenario, who has the result of blood tests available. With 2 minutes remaining in the station directly ask the candidate what they think is the cause for the acute hyperkalaemia in this case. Ask what specific intervention can be used in Intensive Care to treat severe hyperkalaemia. Also ask for the ECG changes associated with hyperkalaemia.

## Actor's Instructions:

You are the nurse looking after Heather, a 72-year-old patient in the acute medical unit. You know she has had very little oral intake for 2 days, and she seems very 'dry'. The GP was concerned about dehydration. Her headache has resolved completely, and she has no signs of any focal neurological deficit, but feels generally weak. She has just been complaining of feeling very thirsty. You had called for assistance from the anaesthetic team for cannulation, but the charge nurse on the ward has just managed to cannulate and has put up 1 litre of intravenous crystalloid (normal saline).

You are concerned as Heather has now become increasingly vague, and the blood test results (samples were sent from her GP surgery) have returned. You can see the highlighted results are abnormal. Your own doctors are off the ward currently.

You have not managed to complete a 12-lead ECG yet, and are preparing to insert a urinary catheter. You are happy to help the doctor by preparing and administering any medicines, but are unsure of doses. The patient has no allergies. You are worried that the patient may deteriorate, and if the doctor doesn't ask for help you should prompt them regarding senior assistance.

**CRITICAL CARE OSCE – Hyperkalaemia**

| Task: | Achieved | Not Achieved |
|---|---|---|
| Introduces self and checks staff name and role | | |
| Briefly clarifies presenting history | | |
| Briefly clarifies past medical history | | |
| Checks allergy status | | |
| Recognises unwell patient and commences ABCDE assessment | | |
| Ensures high flow oxygen administration | | |
| Reviews observations (HR, BP, $SpO_2$, Temperature, blood glucose) | | |
| Reviews blood test results and recognises hyperkalaemia and renal impairment | | |
| Gives a fluid bolus | | |
| Ensures patent IV cannula | | |
| Requests urgent 12-lead ECG checking for changes | | |
| Requests 10ml of intravenous 10% calcium gluconate / calcium chloride | | |
| Requests 10 units intravenous fast-acting insulin in 50ml of 20% dextrose | | |
| Requests nebulized salbutamol (5mg) | | |
| Requests senior assistance | | |
| States monitored / critical care environment required | | |
| Summarises findings and management to examiner | | |
| Understands dehydration and reno-toxic drugs as causes of hyperkalaemia/AKI | | |
| Able to name ECG changes in hyperkalaemia (T tenting, loss of P wave, widening QRS, sine wave, VF) | | |
| States renal replacement therapy may be needed (accept haemofiltration or dialysis) | | |
| | | |
| Examiner's Global Mark | /5 | |
| Actor / Helper's Global Mark | /5 | |
| Total Station Mark | /30 | |

## Learning Points

- The ECG changes in hyperkalaemia are classically described in a stepwise fashion with increasing serum concentrations: tall tented T waves, loss of P waves, widening QRS to the point of 'sine wave pattern', degenerating into ventricular fibrillation.

- Hyperkalaemia is a medical emergency. Increasing concentrations of potassium ions affect the electrochemical stability of the myocardial cell membrane and subsequent action potentials. The acute treatment of hyperkalaemia is designed to 'stabilise' the membrane by redressing this imbalance. Calcium ions are particularly important as an 'antidote' to hyperkalaemia.

- Acute treatment measures may not be enough to allow a sustained reduction in serum potassium concentration (the treatments in this scenario do not eliminate potassium from the body). Treatments for refractory hyperkalaemia include intravenous fluid therapy (and subsequent diuresis), potassium-losing diuretics (furosemide), calcium resonium, and renal replacement therapy (dialysis and haemofiltration).

# CRITICAL CARE OSCE - Diabetic Ketoacidosis

## Candidate's Instructions:

You are a Foundation Year 1 doctor working in the Emergency Department. A 19 year old male called Matthew has been brought in by ambulance after his parents found him drowsy and unwell at his university accommodation.

Please assess the patient and initiate any necessary treatment.

After 6 minutes the examiner will stop you and ask you to summarise back your findings, suggest your management plan and answer some direct questions.

## Examiner's Instructions:

The candidate is a Foundation Year 1 doctor working in the Emergency Department. They have been asked to assess a 19 year old male patient who has been found drowsy and unwell by his parents at his university accommodation.

They will be expected to conduct an A-E assessment which will reveal the following:

A: Patent, no added sounds
B: RR 32, kussmaul respiration, SpO2 98% in air, clear breath sounds throughout
C: HR 125, BP 100/70, cool peripheries, CRT 4s
D: Responds to voice, BM 22mmol/L, no focal neurological deficit, pupils equal and reactive
E: Ketotic breath, no rashes or meningism, no signs of head injury

The candidate should recognise physical signs suggestive of hypovolaemia in the context of a raised plasma glucose and perform a blood gas ABG and urinalysis to confirm the diagnosis of diabetic ketoacidosis.

They should initiate appropriate volume resuscitation and intravenous insulin therapy as well as calling for senior help.

With 2 minutes remaining in the station, ask for a summary of the case and get the candidate to outline the management priorities in the initial hours after presentation. Ask further about the potential electrolyte disturbance which they must be particularly aware of when managing DKA.

## Actor's Instructions:

You are an experienced ED staff nurse working in the resuscitation room. You have just taken handover from an ambulance crew who have brought in Matthew, a 19 year old male found drowsy and unwell in his university accommodation by his parents. According to the crew, Matthew is usually very fit and healthy, but his parents say he does look like he has lost quite a lot of weight since they dropped him off at the start of term.

An F1 doctor in the department will come and assess the patient - you should direct them to the simulation mannequin in order to do this.

They should perform an A-E assessment and you are able to assist with application of monitoring, IV cannulation, preparation of IV fluids and administration of any medication they wish to prescribe.

On arrival in the department, the patient was complaining that he needed to pass urine urgently. You noted that his urine volume was very high and managed to collect a sample for urine dipstick. You should show the doctor the results if they ask for them:

| | |
|---|---|
| **pH** | **5.5** |
| **glucose** | **+++** |
| **Ketones** | **+++** |
| **Leukocytes** | **+** |
| **Protein** | **-** |
| **Nitrites** | **-** |

You are also trained and able to perform a blood gas should the doctor ask for one. The results are as follows:

| | |
|---|---|
| **pH** | **7.01** |
| **pCO2** | **2.8 kPa** |
| **PO2** | **45.6 kPa (on 10L O2 via NRB mask)** |
| **B.E.** | **-16.5** |
| **lactate** | **2.8mmol/L** |
| **HCO3-** | **8.1mmol/L** |

**CRITICAL CARE OSCE - Diabetic Ketoacidosis**

| Task: | Achieved | Not Achieved |
|---|---|---|
| Introduces self and seeks consent to examine | | |
| Applies high flow O2 (10-15L via non rebreath mask) | | |
| Performs an ABCDE assessment | | |
| Asks for application of monitoring (ECG/SpO2/NIBP) | | |
| Inserts/asks for widebore IV cannula (18-16g/green or grey) | | |
| Asks for bloods to be sent (FBC/U&Es/CRP/LFTs/glucose) | | |
| Initiates fluid resuscitation (1L N. Saline/Hartmann's) | | |
| Indicates rapid administration of fluid/'stat' | | |
| Checks blood glucose | | |
| Recognises hyperglycaemia | | |
| Asks for ABG | | |
| Recognises severe metabolic acidosis with partial respiratory compensation | | |
| Asks for urinalysis | | |
| Recognises glycosuria and ketonuria | | |
| Verbalises diagnosis of diabetic ketoacidosis | | |
| Initiates intravenous insulin therapy (e.g. Actrapid 6 units/hr) | | |
| Asks to escalate for senior help (ED/Medical/ICU SpR) | | |
| Summarises case clearly and accurately to examiner | | |
| Identifies management priorities (rapid correction of hypovolaemia/gradual correction of blood sugar and acid base status | | |
| Aware of need to monitor and replace potassium | | |
| Examiner's Global Mark | /5 | |
| Actor / Helper's Global Mark | /5 | |
| Total Station Mark | /30 | |

## Learning Points

- The diagnosis of diabetic ketoacidosis is made by the presence of
  Raised capillary glucose (>11mmol/L)
  Raised capillary ketones (>3mmol/l or urinary ketones > ++ on urine dipstick)
  pH < 7.3 and or bicarbonate < 15mmol/L

- The initial, emergency management of this condition is focused on the correction of hypovolaemia. Rapid administration of 1L of IV crystalloid is appropriate followed by reassessment and ongoing fluid administration. The correction of hyperglycaemia should be gradual and is based on a 'fixed rate intravenous insulin infusion' - typically starting with 0.1units/kg/hr of actrapid. The insulin is used to stop ketogenesis and so falling ketones and not falling BMs are what need to be monitored.

- Potassium replacement is a vitally important part of managing DKA. After the first litre of fluid is rapidly administered, it is typical for the next 2 litres each to be given over 2 hours with 40mmol potassium in each bag. The serum potassium must of course be checked regularly!

# CRITICAL CARE OSCE - Infective exacerbation of COPD

## Candidate's Instructions:

You are the Foundation Year1 doctor on your ICU rotation. You have been sent by your registrar to make a preliminary assessment of Alan, a 67 year old man with a history of COPD who is a frequent attender to the Emergency Department. He has been brought in by ambulance today with severe shortness of breath.

You are required to assess the patient and initiate any appropriate management. You will have an ED nurse present to assist you.

After 6 minutes the examiner will stop you and ask you to summarise back your findings, suggest your management plan and answer some direct questions.

## Examiner's Instructions:

The candidate is a Foundation Year 1 doctor on their ICU rotation. They are attending the Emergency Department ahead of their registrar to make an initial assessment of Alan, a frequent hospital attender with a history of severe COPD on home nebulisation. He has never been admitted to intensive care before.

Today he has presented with what seems like an infective exacerbation and the candidate will be expected to take a focused history, examine the patient and initiate appropriate therapy.

His initial observations are as follows:

| | |
|---|---|
| RR | 34 |
| SpO2 | 82% on 2L oxygen via nasal cannula |
| HR | 120 (sinus tachycardia) |
| BP | 153/81 |
| Temp | 38.2 degrees |

He is alert, short of breath with widespread wheeze throughout both lung fields.

Towards the end of the station you should present the candidate with the following blood gas results:

| | |
|---|---|
| pH | 7.23 |
| PO2 | 7.4 |
| PCO2 | 8.9 |
| HCO3- | 31.2 |
| lactate | 1.8 |
| Hb | 162 |

Ask them to comment on the arterial blood gas and ask what further treatment options they should consider.

## Actor's Instructions:

You are an experienced ED nurse working in the resuscitation room. Alan is a 67 year old male with severe COPD who is a frequent attender to hospital. he has presented today with acute shortness of breath and low oxygen saturations. After a brief assessment by an ED doctor he has been moved to resus and referred for critical care review. You have applied oxygen via nasal cannula - you are careful not to give high flow oxygen in case this causes retention of carbon dioxide.

The Foundation Year1 doctor from intensive care has come to assess the patient in resus. You should direct them to the simulation mannequin in order to do this.

On initial assessment, the candidate will find:

**A:** Patent, talking in short sentences
**B:** RR 34, SpO2 82% on 2L nasal O2, widespread wheeze throughout lung fields
**C:** Warm peripheries, bounding pulses, HR 120, BP 153/81
**D:** Alert, BM 6.5, pupils equal and reactive, no focal neurological deficit
**E:** Soft calves, Temp 38.2, other examination unremarkable

They may ask you to increase the inspired oxygen concentration as the saturations are low. You should be initially resistant to this idea, but will be persuaded if the candidate explains clearly the importance of treating hypoxia.

The candidate should ask you to administer nebulisers, steroids and antibiotics, all of which you are able to do. If the candidate asks for intravenous treatment with magnesium sulphate or aminophylline, you will say that you need to ask a more senior colleague to assist you with preparation.

**CRITICAL CARE OSCE - Infective exacerbation of COPD**

| Task: | Achieved | Not Achieved |
|---|---|---|
| Introduces self & establishes rapport | | |
| Takes a focused history from the patient including PMHx/DHx/SHx | | |
| Asks about changes in sputum production | | |
| Establishes patient is on home nebulisers | | |
| Asks about previous ICU admissions | | |
| Asks about exercise tolerance | | |
| Performs an ABCDE assessment | | |
| Increases FiO2 (accept high flow O2 via non-rebreath or venturi 35%-60%) | | |
| Provides adequate explanation to nurse for increasing FiO2 | | |
| Asks for back to back salbutamol nebulisation (2.5-5mg) | | |
| Asks for ipratropium bromide nebuliser (500mcg) | | |
| Asks for oral/IV steroids | | |
| Inserts IV cannula and sends bloods including blood cultures | | |
| Asks for antibiotics (accept consult trust antibiotic guidelines on infective exacerbation of COPD) | | |
| States would do an arterial blood gas and chest X-ray | | |
| Tells nurse they will escalate to seniors | | |
| Gives an IV fluid bolus (accept 500ml-1L crystalloid) | | |
| Summarises findings and management back to examiner | | |
| Correctly interprets ABG (acute on chronic type II respiratory failure with respiratory acidosis) | | |
| Identifies NIV or intubation and ventilation as treatments for severe respiratory failure | | |
| | | |
| Examiner's Global Mark | /5 | |
| Actor / Helper's Global Mark | /5 | |
| Total Station Mark | /30 | |

## Learning Points

- COPD is a progressive and life-limiting condition in which an exacerbation precipitated by respiratory tract infection can lead to a rapid deterioration in respiratory function. Common causative organisms are bacteria such as Pneumococcus and Haemophilus, and viruses such as influenza, rhinovirus and respiratory syncytial virus.

- A proportion of patients with COPD have chronic carbon dioxide retention (with associated renal retention of bicarbonate ions). A small proportion of these patients may become desensitised to a high arterial PCO2 and rely to some extent on a degree of hypoxia to stimulate their respiratory centres - the 'hypoxic drive'. It is important to understand that these patients are in the minority! In the acute setting, hypoxaemia should be treated with a high inspired oxygen concentration and every patient should have regular clinical review to look for deterioration. It is appropriate to prescribe targeted oxygen therapy, aiming for an SpO2 of 88-92% for patients with chronic hypoxaemia.

- Decompensated chronic respiratory failure, as is presented in this case, is associated with hypoxaemia and a respiratory acidosis. Non-invasive ventilation (NIV) usually in the form of Bi-level Positive Airway Pressure (BiPAP) is delivered via a tight fitting face mask. The machine provides pressure support to breaths triggered by the patient, aiming to increase the tidal volume and improve gas exchange. If successful, NIV can help prevent deterioration and avoid the need for intubation and invasive mechanical ventilation.

# CRITICAL CARE OSCE – Complete heart block

## Candidate's Instructions:

You are a Foundation Year 1 on your ICU placement. You have been asked to review a patient by the critical care outreach sister. Simon is an 82-year-old patient who was admitted after suffering a myocardial infarction 2 days ago.

He has had increasingly frequent episodes of dizziness, and is now back in bed after an episode of syncope. He is drowsy and unable to give much history. The critical care sister is present and able to help you in your assessment and treatment of the patient.

After 6 minutes the examiner will stop you and ask you to summarise back your findings, suggest your management plan and answer some direct questions.

**You are given the below ECG for the patient:**

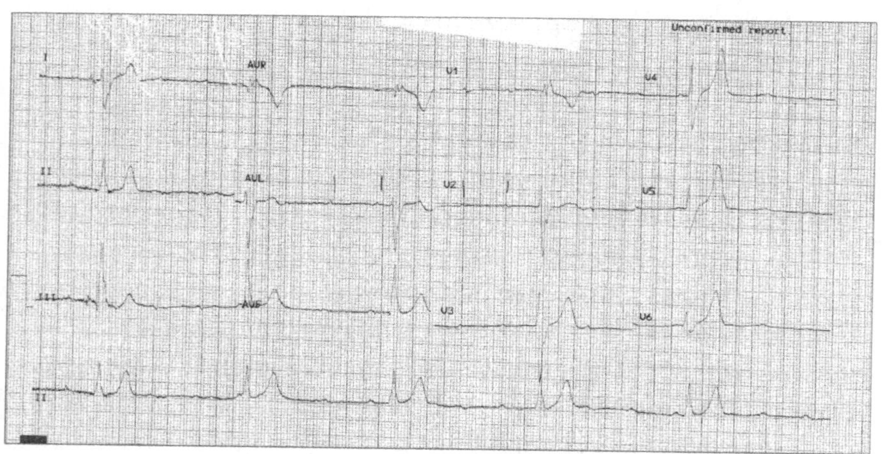

## Examiner's Instructions:

Simon is an 82 year old patient who has a history of ischaemic heart disease related to long term hypertension. He has no valvular disease. He was admitted 2 days ago after an acute myocardial infarction (requiring a single right coronary artery stent) and has now developed complete heart block. He has had an episode of syncope on the coronary care unit. The ECG provided reveals complete heart block, and this is persistent, requiring treatment. He has no allergies.

The candidate is required to assess the situation and offer treatment with the assistance of the critical care outreach sister. Two key aspects of this station are to initiate appropriate monitoring and specifically request assistance from the cardiology team (this will not be immediately available).

The candidate would be expected to progress through the acute management of the patient in an ABCDE fashion, including specific pharmacological management of a bradyarrhythmia (atropine).

With 2 minutes remaining stop the candidate and ask them to summarise their findings. If not offered the candidate should also be asked directly about the use of external cardiac pacing at the end of the station.

## Actor's Instructions:

You are the critical care outreach sister, and have been helping the ward staff on the coronary care unit. The unit is very busy and the cardiology team have just rushed off to the percutaneous intervention suite with another patient.

Simon is an 82-year-old patient who has been recovering well after a myocardial infarction 2 days ago. He required a single stent to his right coronary artery, and was due for discharge from the coronary care unit later today. He has had episodes of dizziness when mobilising over the last 2 hours and a syncopal episode a few minutes ago. He regained consciousness after less than 30 seconds, and has been helped back into bed. He looks a little pale, and is disorientated but calm.

You have completed a 12-lead ECG that you think is abnormal (although you are not confident of the rhythm and require the candidate to check it). You have inserted a cannula and are administering oxygen, but have not attached monitoring yet. When monitoring is attached it reveals a regular heart rate of 35 beats per minute, blood pressure of 95/52 mmHg, $SpO_2$ of 99%, and respiratory rate of 19 breaths per minute. Initial atropine treatment should be requested – but is not effective after a single dose and you would like to know what other options are available for treatment.

**CRITICAL CARE OSCE – Complete heart block**

| Task: | Achieved | Not Achieved |
|---|---|---|
| Introduces self and checks name and role of nurse | | |
| Briefly clarifies presenting history | | |
| Briefly clarifies past medical history | | |
| Makes initial assessment using an ABCDE approach | | |
| Ensures high flow oxygen administration | | |
| Requests monitoring (in particular ECG, BP, $SpO_2$) | | |
| Requests cardiac arrest trolley | | |
| States would attach defibrillator pads | | |
| Reviews current treatment / investigations (including electrolytes) | | |
| Ensures patent IV cannula | | |
| Reviews 12-lead ECG | | |
| Identifies complete heart block | | |
| Requests cardiology team / senior assistance / medical emergency team (MET) call | | |
| Checks allergy status | | |
| Requests atropine IV 500 micrograms bolus | | |
| Indicates need for large IV flush with normal saline after atropine dose | | |
| Indicates potential requirement for further atropine doses to a maximum dose of atropine (3mg) | | |
| Aware of alternative pharmacological therapy for bradyarrhythmia (isoprenaline, adrenaline) | | |
| Summarises finds to examiner | | |
| Indicates potential need for transcutaneous pacing | | |
| | | |
| Examiner's Global Mark | /5 | |
| Actor / Helper's Global Mark | /5 | |
| Total Station Mark | /30 | |

## Learning Points

- The UK Resuscitation Council produces Advanced Life Support (ALS) algorithms for the management of a range of malignant arrhythmias and cardiac arrest. They allow multidisciplinary teams to work through specific steps to ensure standardised and timely treatment.

- In stressful situations the recollection of specific drugs, doses, and defibrillator energy settings may be fallible. Cognitive aids are tools that allow individuals to access relevant information quickly. These include printed algorithms and smartphone applications, and are an essential part of modern practice.

- The pattern of coronary arterial supply to structures in the heart is often predictable. A knowledge of which structure ischaemia may affect is useful to help predict resultant complications. The atrioventricular node is commonly supplied by the right coronary artery, which is relevant in this scenario.

# CRITICAL CARE OSCE - Anaphylaxis

## Candidate's Instructions:

You are a Foundation Year 1 on the orthopaedic ward.

A staff nurse asks you to see Dan, a 28 year old awaiting wash-out of an infected elbow effusion. He complained of feeling unwell as the nurse was completing her drug rounds. Please assess him, state your diagnosis and initiate appropriate management.

After 6 minutes the examiner will stop you and ask you to summarise back your findings, suggest your management plan and answer some direct questions.

## Examiner's Instructions:

Dan is a 28 year old awaiting wash-out of an infected elbow effusion. He began feeling unwell shortly after an infusion of Flucloxacillin commenced.

The candidate should perform an A to E assessment of a mannequin, where they should initially note lip swelling, mild wheeze, a modest tachycardia and hypotension

The patient will go on to show signs of deterioration - worsening airway oedema, worsening wheeze, shock and rash as a late sign.

They should declare an emergency, summon appropriate help, and administer IM adrenaline at the correct dose.

With 2 minutes remaining ask the candidate to summarise the case, the management so far, and next steps, including the need for ICU admission.

## Assistant's Instructions:

You are a staff nurse who has asked the candidate to see Dan, a 28 year old awaiting wash -out of an infected elbow effusion. He complained of feeling unwell as you were completing your drug rounds - he feels light headed, anxious and "just not right."

Direct the candidate to make an assessment of the Mannequin. Initial findings will be as follows;

**A**: Talking in full sentences, but complaining his lips feel "puffy".
**B**: RR 24, SpO2 96% on air, central trachea, equal chest expansion, resonant percussion note throughout, mild bilateral wheeze.
**C**: Warm peripheries, central and capillary refill less than 2 seconds, regular radial pulse rate of 110/min, blood pressure 90/50.
**D**: Alert/GCS 15. Pupils 3mm, equal and reactive, BM 5
**E**: Temperature 36.7. An infusion of 2g of Flucloxacillin is in progress. No rash, but face and chest look flushed.

If the candidate asks for further history, the patient is normally fit and well, has no known allergies, and was admitted this morning with an infected elbow infusion. You have just commenced his first dose of IV flucloxacillin.

His last set of observations before complaining of feeling unwell showed a RR of 16, SpO2 of 99% on air, heart rate of 90 and blood pressure of 115/80.

Following the initial assessment the candidate may ask you to perform certain tasks or administer medications. Please state that you are happy to do so, but ask specifically for drug doses and route of administration.

We would expect them to request;

**Adrenaline**: This should be given as 0.5mL of 1:1000 adrenaline **IM**, and can be repeated if needed every 5 minutes.

If they don't volunteer a specific dose and route for adrenaline, please show them both the 1:1000 and 1:10 000 Minijets and ask them to tell you which one to give and via which route.
**Oxygen**: 15L via a Non-Rebreathe Mask.
**IV fluids:** 500 or 1000ml of crystalloid, either Normal Saline or Hartmanns Solution.
**Chlorphenamine: 10mg IV.**
**Hydrocortisone: 200mg IV.**

The patient should complain of feeling more unwell and on re-assessment the candidate will find:

**A**: Stridor, struggling to speak
**B**: Widespread wheeze, reduced air entry
**C: HR 140, BP 60/30**
**D: Eye opening to voice**
**E**: Lip and tongue swelling, urticarial rash over chest wall

If they have not already done so, we would expect them to summon urgent help and administer or repeat IM adrenaline, as well as request any of the measures above which are outstanding.

After a second appropriate dose of IM adrenaline, tell the candidate that the patient is showing signs of improvement.

*NB: If high dose adrenaline (0.5-1mg) is wrongly administered intravenously, the patient should should develop short lived but profound tachycardia (>180) and hypertension (200/110).*

**CRITICAL CARE OSCE - Anaphylaxis**

| Task: | Achieved | Not Achieved |
|---|---|---|
| Introduces self to patient | | |
| Briefly clarifies history of acute problem | | |
| Briefly clarifies past medical and drug history | | |
| Enquires about allergy status | | |
| Performs ABCDE assessment | | |
| Picks up on clinical signs - lip swelling, wheeze, hypotension, tachycardia, flushing/rash | | |
| Recognises and verbalises diagnosis of anaphylaxis | | |
| Escalates early and calls for appropriate help eg 2222 , senior doctor/ anaesthetist | | |
| Administers IM adrenaline 500mcg | | |
| Gives 10-15L of Oxygen using non-rebreathe mask | | |
| Seeks precipitants - asks patient, nursing staff, looks at drug chart | | |
| Stops IV Flucloxacillin immediately | | |
| Gives 500-1000ml Crystalloid bolus | | |
| Requests 200mg IV Hydrocortisone | | |
| Requests 10mg IV Chlorphenamine | | |
| Recognises deterioration and repeats ABCDE assessment | | |
| States the need to repeat IM adrenaline after 5 minutes | | |
| Summarises case to examiner | | |
| Aware of need for ongoing treatment on ICU | | |
| Aware of need for drug error incident reporting | | |
| | | |
| Examiner's Global Mark | /5 | |
| Actor / Helper's Global Mark | /5 | |
| Total Station Mark | /30 | |

## Learning Points

- Anaphylaxis is a severe, life-threatening, systemic hypersensitivity reaction. It causes a rapidly evolving compromise of the airway, breathing and circulation. Skin changes, e.g. urticarial rash, flushing or mucosal swelling, are absent in 20% of cases.

- The most important treatment is adrenaline, which treats vasodilatation and bronchoconstriction, and also stabilises mast cells. The correct adult dose is 0.5ml of 1:1000 (500mcg) administered IM. The ideal site of administration is the middle third of the thigh, along the anterolateral border.

- Mast Cell Tryptase levels confirm a diagnosis of anaphylaxis. Ideally 3 samples should be taken: during resuscitation; 1-2 hours after the onset of symptoms; and 24 hours later.

# CRITICAL CARE OSCE - TRAUMA

## Candidate's Instructions:

A 26 year old male has been admitted to the Emergency Department following a road traffic accident (RTA). He has a C-spine collar in situ.

You are the Foundation Year1 doctor in the ED and have been tasked with performing the primary survey.

After 6 minutes the examiner will stop you and ask you to summarise back your findings, suggest your management plan and answer some direct questions.

## Examiner's Instructions:

A 26 year old male has been brought into the ED having been involved in a road traffic accident. The man already has a C-spine collar fitted. He complains of left sided chest pain and has a haemothorax.

The Foundation Year1 doctor in the ED team has been asked to take perform the primary survey and feedback their findings to the team leader. The relevant findings are as follows:

- The airway is patent with no blood/debris in the mouth
- The patient's oxygen saturations are 94% on air (and 98% on 15L/min of oxygen)
- The respiratory rate is 26/min
- There is left chest bruising
- Chest expansion is reduced on the left
- The left lower zone has a stony dull percussion note with reduced breath sounds
- **Heart sounds are normal**
- Pulse is 100/min. Blood pressure is 110/80.
- There are no external signs of abdominal, pelvic or limb trauma
- **The GCS is E4 V5 M6**
- Pupils are equal and reactive to light
- **Glucose is 7.0 mmol/L**
- **Temperature is 36.5 C**
- The CXR is not performed by the end of the examination

After the primary survey is complete (or 6 minutes has elapsed), ask the candidate to summarise their findings and formulate a management plan.

## Actor's Instructions:

You are a 26 year old male who has been brought into the ED having been involved in an RTA. You vaguely remember what happened and can recall skidding to avoid a dog in the road. You had a seatbelt on and were travelling at approximately 30mph. The steering wheel and side airbags have both deployed and you are aware that they seemed to have hit you in the chest.

The paramedics arrived within minutes and helped you out of the car and fitted a C-spine collar at scene and transported you on a hard board. You now have some discomfort in the left side of your chest. Your breathing feels slightly different but you are able to talk in full sentences and are not bringing up any blood or sputum. You have no other pain specifically in your abdomen, pelvis or lower limbs and are able to move all four limbs fully.

You are otherwise fit and well, have no allergies and last ate over 6 hours ago.

**CRITICAL CARE OSCE - Trauma**

| Task: | Achieved | Not Achieved |
|---|---|---|
| Introduces self and applies personal protection equipment – gloves, gown and glasses. | | |
| Assesses airway by speaking to the patient and asking him to open his mouth | | |
| Records $SpO_2$ and applies oxygen via a facemask | | |
| Inspects the chest for any injuries | | |
| Counts respiratory rate | | |
| Looks for chest expansion | | |
| Checks percussion note | | |
| Listens for breath sounds in all zones and on both sides | | |
| Auscultates heart sounds | | |
| Palpates pulses centrally | | |
| Measures blood pressure | | |
| Inserts 2 large bore IV devices and draws blood for baseline laboratory tests | | |
| Assesses GCS | | |
| Checks pupillary light reflex | | |
| Checks blood glucose | | |
| Exposes patient and looks for abdominal, pelvic and limb abnormalities | | |
| Checks the patient's temperature | | |
| Diagnoses probable haemothorax and orders CXR | | |
| Summarises findings back to the examiner | | |
| Identifies correct treatment of surgical chest drainage | | |
| | | |
| Examiner's Global Mark | /5 | |
| Actor / Helper's Global Mark | /5 | |
| Total Station Mark | /30 | |

## Learning Points

- Have a structured approach to the primary survey:

  Airway maintenance with cervical spine protection
  Breathing and ventilation
  Circulation with haemorrhage control
  Disability (neurological status)
  Exposure and environmental control (expose the patient but avoid hypothermia)

- Once life-threatening injuries have been identified, address them before moving on. Once an intervention has been made (no matter how small) remember to reassess and check the effect of that intervention in a timely manner.

- Effective communication is crucial – feedback findings to the team leader so that ongoing care can be planned effectively.

# CRITICAL CARE OSCE - Narrow Complex Tachycardia

## Candidate's Instructions:

Sarah is a 31 year old female who has presented to the emergency department complaining of a 1 hour history of palpitations after a night out with her friends.

You are the Foundation Year1 doctor in the ED and have been tasked with performing the primary survey.

After 6 minutes the examiner will stop you and ask you to summarise back your findings, suggest your management plan and answer some direct questions.

## Examiner's Instructions:

Sarah is a 31 year old female with a past medical history of supraventricular tachycardia. She has had several previous attendances at the emergency department where she has needed treatment with adenosine and once received a DC shock. She is awaiting follow up with her cardiology team who are considering her for an ablation.

Today she has presented after having had a night out with friends drinking alcohol. She is stable initially with no adverse signs (Alert, HR 190, BP 100/60, SpO2 99% on air, RR 18). The candidate will be expected to perform an initial A-E assessment, establish IV access and connect to cardiac monitoring.

After 5 minutes, the patient will start to complain of chest tightness and shortness of breath. The candidate will be expected to consider DC cardioversion and call for senior help. Encourage the candidate to talk you through their findings as they go along.

With 2 minutes remaining ask the candidate to summarise the case, the management so far, and next steps, including the need for DC Cardioversion and early escalation to cardiology.

## Actor's Instructions:

You are Sarah, a 31 year old female with a past medical history of supraventricular tachycardia. You woke up this morning after a night out with friends with the feeling of your heart racing in your chest, which you recognise as an SVT. You have come in to your local emergency department for treatment.

You are otherwise fit and well and the only medication you take is the oral contraceptive pill. You have no drug allergies. You smoke socially when you are out and admit to binge drinking once a fortnight when you may have up to 20 units in one evening. You have never used recreational drugs.

At the moment you are feeling ok, provided you sit still. A few minutes into the assessment by the doctor you begin to feel some tightness in your chest and it becomes more difficult to breath, which scares you. You remember the last time this happened that they had to give your heart an electric shock, which was horrible. You really don't want this to happen again, but you will cooperate with whatever the doctor thinks is best.

**CRITICAL CARE OSCE - Narrow Complex Tachycardia**

| Task: | Achieved | Not Achieved |
|---|---|---|
| Introduces self & establishes rapport with patient | | |
| Applies high flow oxygen during assessment | | |
| Takes a brief, focused history from the patient | | |
| Assesses the Airway – by talking to the patient | | |
| Assesses breathing (RR/inspection/palpation/auscultation) | | |
| Assess circulation (palpates pulse/auscultates heart/asks for BP) | | |
| Connects to monitoring (3 lead ECG/SpO2/NIBP) | | |
| Assesses heart rhythm on monitor | | |
| Identifies regular narrow complex tachycardia | | |
| Correctly identifies the absence of adverse signs | | |
| Suggests vagal manouvres | | |
| Inserts an IV cannula and draws blood samples | | |
| Suggests adenosine | | |
| Assesses Disability (comments on AVPU/asks for BM) | | |
| Assesses Exposure (looks for rashes/blood loss/palpates for calf swelling) | | |
| Recognises deterioration and reassesses | | |
| Asks for senior help | | |
| Summarises findings back to examiner | | |
| Recognises adverse features and the need for possible DC cardioversion | | |
| Recognises need for sedation with Anaesthetic support | | |
| | | |
| Examiner's Global Mark | /5 | |
| Actor / Helper's Global Mark | /5 | |
| Total Station Mark | /30 | |

## Learning Points

- Narrow complex tachycardias are a common emergency presentation, which may affect young people. It is important to make a methodical ABCDE assessment, paying particular attention to signs of physiological compromise and following the ALS tachyarrhythmia algorithm. The four adverse features to check for are shock, syncope, myocardial ischemia and heart failure. These features are the same for tachy and brady arrhythmias, which can severely compromise the cardiac output.

- Regular Narrow complex tachycardia without compromise can be treated with vagal manoeuvres or adenosine. Adenosine is a short acting agent which blocks the atrioventricular node. It can make patients feel unwell with a sense of chest heaviness, so counsel them appropriately before administration.

- A compromised patient with any tachyarrhythmia needs DC cardioversion. To perform this the patient will need sedation or general anaesthesia. You should ensure you urgently seek help from your seniors and inform the on call Anaesthetist.

# CRITICAL CARE OSCE - Acute severe asthma

## Candidate's Instructions:

Carl is a 28-year-old man with a history of asthma who has presented to the Emergency Department with difficulty breathing.

You are a Foundation Year 1 doctor on your anaesthetics rotation and you have been asked to assess him.

After 6 minutes the examiner will stop you and ask you to summarise back your findings, suggest your management plan and answer some direct questions.

## Examiner's Instructions:

Carl is a 28-year-old man who has presented to the ED acutely short of breath.

He has a history of asthma that has required hospitalisation on numerous occasions. 2 years ago he was admitted to ICU following an acute exacerbation. He has been unwell for the last 2 hours with worsening wheeze. He has no pain, fever or cough. He usually takes nebulisers and Monteleukast for his asthma, but has a history of relatively poor compliance with this treatments. He has no allergies.

Carl is unwell, can barely manage to finish a sentence and has the following observations; $SpO_2$ 94% on air, respiratory rate of 35, HR of 120/min regular, a PEFR of 200L/min and on auscultation has widespread polyphonic wheeze. His blood pressure is 130/70.

With 2 minutes remaining stop the candidate and ask them to summarise their findings and subsequent management plan.

## Actor's Instructions:

You are a 28-year-old man who has presented to the ED acutely short of breath.

You have a history of poorly controlled asthma and have been admitted to hospital on a number of occasions. 2 years ago you were on a breathing machine in ICU. You take a number of medications including nebulisers and some tablets. You have no allergies. You sometimes forget to take your peak flow reading, but think on a good day it is around 400. You have been fairly well recently, and this attack has some out of the blue. You cannot recall which asthma medications you usually take as when you are well you often forget to take them. You have a history of eczema and hayfever and use medications as and when for these. You smoke socially but never more than 5 per evening.

You feel wheezy and very short of breath, so much so that you are having difficulty finishing sentences. You do not have any cough, fever or chest pain. You are very scared as this attacks feels more severe than others and you are very short of breath.

CRITICAL CARE OSCE - Acute severe asthma

| Task: | Achieved | Not Achieved |
|---|---|---|
| Introduces self & establishes rapport | | |
| Asks about onset and severity of dyspnoea | | |
| Asks about associated features: fever, chest pain, cough. | | |
| Asks about previous asthma history | | |
| Takes a drug and allergy history | | |
| Takes a social history including smoking history | | |
| Counts respiratory rate | | |
| Asks for pulse oximeter and checks pulse rate | | |
| Asks for oxygen to be applied to obtain SpO2 of >94% | | |
| Comments on chest expansion and percussion note – both normal | | |
| Identifies wheeze | | |
| Asks for Peak expiratory flow reading but accepts patient may be too unwell to perform it | | |
| Considers arterial blood gas analysis | | |
| Asks for NIBP | | |
| Elicits concerns from the patient and responds in an appropriate manner | | |
| Summarises the case and identifies features of severe asthma | | |
| Asks for back to back nebulised salbutamol 2.5-5mg | | |
| Asks for a dose of steroids (IV or oral acceptable) | | |
| Escalates early and considers the use of magnesium after senior discussion | | |
| Summarises findings back to the examiner | | |
| | | |
| Examiner's Global Mark | /5 | |
| Actor / Helper's Global Mark | /5 | |
| Total Station Mark | /30 | |

## Learning Points

- Acute severe asthma may be suggested by any one of:
    - PEFR 33-50% best or predicted
    - Respiratory rate ≥ 25/minute
    - Heart rate ≥ 110/min
    - Inability to complete sentences

- The principles of acute treatment are oxygen to target a $SpO_2$ 94-98%, nebulised bronchodilators and steroids. Magnesium may be considered after senior consultation as per the British Thoracic Society guidelines.

- Features of life threatening asthma include a silent chest, exhaustion, a normal (or elevated $pCO_2$) or hypotension and will necessitate referral to the critical care team. Beware a patient with asthma who has been previously admitted to ICU!

# CRITICAL CARE OSCE - SUBARACHNOID HAEMORRHAGE

## Candidate's Instructions:

You are a Foundation Year 1 doctor in the emergency department. You have been asked to assess Maria who is a 57 year old female patient presenting to hospital with an acute onset of severe headache. She has no significant past medical history.

You are a Foundation Year doctor on your Emergency Department placement and you have been asked to assess her.

After 6 minutes the examiner will stop you and ask you to summarise back your findings, suggest your management plan and answer some direct questions.

## Examiner's Instructions:

Maria is a 57 year old female with no past medical history who has been brought in by ambulance with an acute history of severe headache.

The candidate is a Foundation Year doctor in the emergency department who has been asked to make an initial assessment. On arrival in the department the patient is responsive to voice with confused speech. The remaining physiological parameters are within normal limits.

After the initial A-E assessment, the patient's neurological condition will deteriorate and they will begin to show signs of partial airway obstruction requiring a jaw thrust and insertion of an oropharyngeal airway (OPA). The candidate will be expected to maintain airway patency while calling for urgent senior assistance. You should ask them to size and insert the OPA when appropriate. Encourage the candidates to talk through their findings as they go along.

With 2 minutes remaining ask the candidate to summarise the case, the management so far, and next steps, including the need for an urgent CT scan.

## Actor's Instructions:

You are Maria, a 57 year old female who is usually fit and healthy. This morning you developed a very severe and sudden onset headache. Your husband called the ambulance and you were brought to the emergency department.

When you arrive in hospital, you are unable to communicate clearly and your speech is muddled. You are in considerable pain and are lying with your eyes closed, but you open your eyes when somebody talks to you.

You have diet controlled diabetes but otherwise have no medical problems and have never suffered from headaches. You take over the counter multivitamins and have no drug allergies. You are a non smoker and drink a maximum of 4 units of alcohol per week. You work in the local school office twice a week and live with your husband and eldest son.

A short time after the doctor assesses you, you lose consciousness and begin to snore. During this time you are no longer responsive to voice or to painful stimulus.

**CRITICAL CARE OSCE - SUBARACHNOID HAEMORRHAGE**

| Task: | Achieved | Not Achieved |
|---|---|---|
| Introduces self | | |
| Briefly clarifies history of presentation | | |
| Assesses the Airway (by talking to patient) and applies high flow oxygen | | |
| Assesses Breathing (RR/Inspection/palpation/auscultation/SpO2) | | |
| Assesses Circulation (Palpates pulse/CRT/asks for blood pressure) | | |
| Applies monitoring (3 lead ECG/SpO2/NIBP) | | |
| Assesses Disability (AVPU, asks for BM, checks pupillary reaction to light) | | |
| Identifies 'V' on AVPU | | |
| Assesses Exposure (looks for a rash/signs of blood loss/palpates calves) | | |
| Recognises deterioration when patient becomes less responsive/snoring | | |
| Reassesses Airway (look/listen/feel) | | |
| Opens airway appropriately (head tilt, chin lift/jaw thrust) | | |
| Correctly sizes and inserts OP airway | | |
| Reassesses airway after intervention to ensure patency and reapplies oxygen | | |
| Calls for urgent senior support (ED senior/Anaesthetist) | | |
| Repeats brief A-E assessment after deterioration | | |
| Identifies drop in conscious level ('U' on AVPU) | | |
| Summarises findings to examiner | | |
| Can identify Subarachnoid haemorrhage as a differential | | |
| States urgent CT scan will be needed but need for intubation and ventilation prior to scan | | |
| Examiner's Global Mark | /5 | |
| Actor / Helper's Global Mark | /5 | |
| Total Station Mark | /30 | |

## Learning Points

- Subarachnoid haemorrhage is a life threatening emergency that is characterised by acute severe headache with or without a depressed level of consciousness. It should be high on the list of differentials in any patient who presents with an acute headache and requires urgent investigation and treatment. If a subarachnoid haemorrhage is proven on the CT scan, neuroprotective measures such as elevating the head, glycaemic control and maintenance of normocapnia will be undertaken until discussion with neurosurgery confirms the ongoing management.

- Basic airway management is a core skill for all clinicians. It is imperative that you are able to recognise the signs of airway obstruction and utilise simple manoeuvres and adjuncts to maintain a patent airway until senior or specialist help arrives.

- A patient's airway protective reflexes become impaired below a GCS of 8 (P or U on the AVPU scale). Patients who are comatose require urgent assessment by an Anaesthetist and may need to be intubated for airway protection, especially if they need to have a CT scan or be transferred to another hospital.

# CRITICAL CARE OSCE - Severe hyponatraemia

## Candidate's Instructions:

Jeanie is a 76-year-old female who has been admitted to the Emergency Department (ED) after being found slumped in her chair by her daughter. She has lung cancer and had a lobectomy over a year ago. Her last course of chemotherapy was over a month ago.

You are the Foundation Year doctor in the ED and have been asked to perform the initial assessment. Jeanie's daughter is present and can answer any questions and an ED nurse is available to help you. Assess the patient with a view to making a diagnosis and formulate an initial management plan.

After 6 minutes the examiner will stop you and ask you to summarise back your findings, suggest your management plan and answer some direct questions.

## Examiner's Instructions:

Jeanie is a 76-year-old female who has been brought into the ED having been found slumped in her chair at home. She has lung cancer and has been treated with a lobectomy and chemotherapy. She currently takes paracetamol and furosemide only. Jeanie's daughter is present and can answer any questions. There is no history of diabetes, stroke or epilepsy and Jeanie no longer smokes or drinks any alcohol.

The Foundation Year doctor in the ED team has been asked to take perform the initial assessment and formulate a management plan. The relevant findings are as follows:

A: The airway is patent and the patient responds to a question with a confused answer
B: The patient's oxygen saturations are 94% on air
The respiratory rate is 20/min
Respiratory examination is normal
C: Pulse is 100/min. Blood pressure is 110/80.
D: The patient is V on the AVPU scale
There is no external sign of head trauma
Pupils are equal and reactive to light

There is no meningism
All 4 limbs appear to be moving and reflexes are normal
Glucose is 7.0 mmol/L

Temperature is 35.5 C
Sodium is 110 mmol/L on a venous gas. Other parameters are normal.

With 2 minutes remaining ask the candidate to summarise their findings, the management so far, and ask directly about the hyponatraemia.

## Actor's Instructions:

### *Patient:*

You are a 76-year-old female who has been brought into the ED having been found at home. You are confused and don't remember the last few hours. You don't understand what is happening.

### *Daughter:*

You have come into hospital with your mother who you found very unwell and drowsy in her home earlier today when you popped round for a visit. Your mother had a part of her left lung removed a year ago. She completed her 3rd cycle of chemotherapy over a month ago and had been doing quite well, though she has been very fatigued during her treatment. Before all this her mother had always been in good health with no other previous medical problems. She only takes paracetamol occasionally for aches and pains and a water tablet called frusemide which her GP gave her for swollen legs. She is not allergic to anything, is an ex smoker and drinks no alcohol. You are very concerned about how confused your mum seems and are convinced that the cancer must have come back and spread to her brain.

**CRITICAL CARE OSCE - Severe hyponatraemia**

| Task: | Achieved | Not Achieved |
|---|---|---|
| Introduces self to patient + daughter and establishes rapport | | |
| Briefly clarifies history from daughter and patient | | |
| Assesses airway | | |
| Assesses breathing (RR/inspection/palpation/ percussion/auscultation/$SpO_2$) | | |
| Assesses circulation (HR/BP/CRT/3 lead ECG monitoring) | | |
| Assesses conscious level- GCS or AVPU - notes V on AVPU | | |
| Checks for external signs of head trauma | | |
| Checks blood glucose | | |
| Notes that all 4 limbs are moving | | |
| Checks peripheral reflexes including plantar response | | |
| Checks for neck stiffness | | |
| Checks pupillary light reflexes | | |
| Checks temperature | | |
| Identifies hyponatraemia on venous blood gas | | |
| Re Clarifies a medication history | | |
| Explains problem of hyponatraemia | | |
| Deals compassionately with patient and her daughter | | |
| Escalates early to senior colleague | | |
| Summarises case to examiner and presents a differential diagnosis (including SIADH and diuretic induced) | | |
| Outlines treatment plan (correction of hyponatraemia with hypertonic saline in monitored environment) | | |
| Examiner's Global Mark | /5 | |
| Actor / Helper's Global Mark | /5 | |
| Total Station Mark | /30 | |

## Learning Points

- A systematic approach is essential when assessing a patient with an abnormal conscious level - there are numerous potential causes especially in patients with multiple comorbidities and many of which are easily overlooked!

- Hyponatraemia usually has multiple causes with SIADH and drug induced (especially diuretics) the commonest. It is important to know a list of potential causes based upon the patient's fluid status, serum and urinary osmolarities and urinary sodium levels.

- In severe, symptomatic hyponatraemia (as in this case), raising the serum sodium by 4 to 6 mmol/L with hypertonic saline (e.g. 2.7% NaCl, 2ml/kg) should generally reduce symptoms and prevent cerebral herniation. Correction to a 'normal' level can then take place slowly over the next couple of days. Needless to say, senior help is essential!

# Critical Care OSCE - Choking

## Candidate's Instructions:

You are a foundation doctor working in Emergency Department and a staff nurse has asked you to urgently assist with a man who appears to be choking in the waiting room.
After 6 minutes the examiner will stop you and ask you to summarise back your findings, suggest your management plan and answer some direct questions.

## Examiner's Instructions:

The foundation doctor has been called to assist with a man that is choking in the waiting room of the Emergency Department.

The scenario should be conducted using a mannequin. The candidate is required to progress through the ALS choking algorithm with assistance from a helper who will play the role of the nurse in the scenario.

With 2 minutes remaining ask the candidate to summarise their management and ask how the foreign body could be removed after the patient has arrested. As a follow up question, ask the candidate what other means are available for oxygenation should attempts to relive the upper airway obstruction be unsuccessful.

## Actor's Instructions:

You are a nurse in the Emergency Department. You have sought help from one of the Foundation doctors to manage a patient who appears to be choking in the waiting room.

Use the following information to guide the candidate through the station, which should be conducted on a resuscitation mannequin:

The patient is conscious initially and is coughing in order to relieve a partial airway obstruction. The candidate should initially encourage coughing and observe for signs of deterioration.

After a short time, tell the candidate that further coughing efforts are silent and that the patient is showing signs of respiratory distress.

The candidate should deliver back blows and abdominal thrusts in order to relieve the airway obstruction.

Allow the candidate to perform 2 rounds of 5 back blows and 5 abdominal thrusts before informing them that the patient appears to have lost consciousness.

The candidate should then check for signs of life and, having confirmed cardiac arrest, they should summon the arrest team and start basic life support with your assistance.

**CRITICAL CARE OSCE - choking**

| Task: | Achieved | Not Achieved |
|---|---|---|
| Introduces self | | |
| Assesses airway by talking to the patient | | |
| Correctly identifies patient has partial airway obstruction with an effective cough | | |
| Encourages cough | | |
| Recognises complete airway obstruction signified by silent cough | | |
| Identifies patient is deteriorating and acts swiftly | | |
| Calls for help / cardiac arrest call initiated | | |
| Administers back blow before abdominal thrust | | |
| Correctly administers 5 back blows | | |
| Reassesses to see if back blow have cleared airway obstruction | | |
| Recognises need for further treatment when airway obstruction persists | | |
| Correctly administers 5 abdominal thrusts | | |
| Reassesses to see if abdominal thrusts have cleared airway obstruction | | |
| Repeats cycle of back blows and abdominal thrusts while patient remains conscious | | |
| Checks for signs of life when patient appears to lose consciousness | | |
| Diagnoses cardiac arrest and calls arrest team/2222 | | |
| Performs CPR 30:2 with help from nurse | | |
| Proceeds through algorithm swiftly and calmly | | |
| Question 1 - knows that foreign body should only be removed under direct vision/laryngoscopy by appropriately trained person | | |
| Question 2 - knows that a surgical airway is a technique to restore oxygenation in this situation | | |
| | | |
| Examiner's Global Mark | /5 | |
| Actor / Helper's Global Mark | /5 | |
| Total Station Mark | /30 | |

## Learning Points

- Recognising signs of airway obstruction is a crucial skill. Remember, a partially obstructed airway is noisy. This noise is caused by turbulent air flowing past the obstruction e.g. stridor. Most concerning is if the patient with airway obstruction is silent - this means no air is moving and the patient has total airway obstruction. This must be relieved immediately or the patient will quickly go on to have a hypoxic cardiac arrest.

- Never try to manually remove a foreign body in a patient who is choking. An appropriately skilled individual may be able to retrieve the object with suction or forceps under direct vision using a laryngoscope. To do this safely, the patient must be either anaesthetised or unconscious.

- In situations where an airway cannot be established via the mouth or nose, Anaesthetists are trained to access the airway surgically by performing a cricothyroidotomy.

# Critical Care OSCE: Cardiac arrest

## Candidate's instructions:

A 65 year old man admitted with SOB and pleuritic chest pain has collapsed and become unresponsive on the cardiology ward. The nurse at the bedside has shouted for help.

You are the foundation doctor on ward cover and you are the first to attend. Please assess the patient and manage accordingly.

After 6 minutes the examiner will stop you and ask you to summarise back your findings, suggest your management plan and answer some direct questions.

## Examiner's Instructions:

A 65 year old man admitted with SOB and pleuritic chest pain has collapsed on the cardiology ward. The nurse at the bedside has shouted for help. The candidate is the foundation doctor on the ward and is the first to attend.

They are expected to confirm cardiac arrest and put out a cardiac arrest call. They should identify and initial rhythm of VF on the defibrillator and deliver a shock appropriately. Following one shock and 2mins of CPR the rhythm will switch to PEA. Following administration of adrenaline and further 2mins of CPR there is return of spontaneous circulation (ROSC).

Ask the candidate to identify the reversible causes of cardiac arrest (4 Hs & 4 Ts) and which is the most likely in this case.

## Actor's Instructions:

You are the nurse on the cardiology ward. Your patient, Adam is a 65 year old man admitted with SOB and pleuritic chest pain, has just collapsed

The candidate will check for signs of life – inform them there is no pulse or breathing

The candidate will perform CPR on the mannequin

Connect the defibrillator when asked

Assist with ventilation if asked by the candidate

At the first rhythm check the defibrillator should show VF

After one shock and 2 minutes CPR, the defibrillator should show a rate of 120bpm with no pulse (PEA)

After 1mg adrenaline and a further 2 minutes CPR, the rhythm is a sinus tachycardia and there is a palpable carotid pulse indicating ROSC.

**Critical Care OSCE: Cardiac Arrest**

| Task: | Achieved | Not Achieved |
|---|---|---|
| Looks for danger | | |
| Checks patient for response | | |
| Look, listens and feels for breathing for <10 sec | | |
| Simultaneously feels carotid <10 sec | | |
| Confirms cardiac arrest and calls for resuscitation team (2222) | | |
| Starts chest compressions at 100-120/min at depth of 5-6cm | | |
| Asks nurse to attach defibrillator pads whilst continuing CPR | | |
| Asks nurse to ventilate patient with a bag valve mask (30:2) | | |
| Pauses CPR to assess rhythm briefly | | |
| Correctly identifies VF | | |
| Charges defibrillator | | |
| Clear command to stand clear and remove oxygen | | |
| Delivers shock safely | | |
| Resume CPR immediately for 2 mins then reassess | | |
| Identifies PEA and administers adrenaline 1mg IV/IO immediately | | |
| Continues CPR for 2 mins then reassess | | |
| Identifies sinus rhythm Checks for pulse to confirm ROSC | | |
| Summarises findings to examiner | | |
| Identifies reversible causes with 'thrombus' most likely | | |
| | | |
| Examiner's Global Mark | /5 | |
| Actor / Helper's Global Mark | /5 | |
| Total Station Mark | /30 | |

## Learning Points:

- It is important to be able to deliver high quality chest compressions with minimal interruptions as this can significantly influence outcome. Performing compressions is tiring so no one person should ever do more than one cycle in a row where personnel allow for regular rotation. A key time to remember this is once the rhythm has been confirmed as shockable chest compressions should be restarted and continue while the defibrillator is charging.

- Look for reversible causes and treat early – remember 4H's and 4T's of Hypoxia, Hypovolaemia, Hypo/Hyper electrolytaemia, hypothermia and Tension pneumothorax, tamponade, Toxins and Thrombus. Each cause should be considered and excluded fully.

- Use an ABCDE approach immediately following ROSC and ensure necessary investigations are carried out to identify and treat precipitating causes. High quality of care must be sustained before safe transfer to critical care facility.

# CRITICAL CARE OSCE - Spinal cord injury

## Candidate's Instructions:

Daniel is a 25-year-old man who was knocked off his bike and landed on his back. He has been brought to the emergency department and is complaining that he can't move his legs.

You are a Foundation Year doctor and have been asked to finish the primary survey. Your senior colleague has already assessed Daniel's airway and breathing. He appears to have a diaphragmatic breathing pattern and respiratory rate of 25. Continue the primary survey from 'C' .

After 6 minutes the examiner will stop you and ask you to summarise back your findings, suggest your management plan and answer some direct questions.

## Examiner's Instructions:

Daniel is a 25-year-old man who was knocked off his bike and landed on his back. He has been brought to the emergency department and is complaining that he can't move his legs. His airway and breathing have already been assessed. He has a diaphragmatic breathing pattern and respiratory rate of 25. A C-spine collar is already in situ.

The candidate should continue the primary survey.

The clinical findings are as follows:

- Heart rate of 40/min
- Blood pressure of 80/50
- GCS 15
- Pupils equal and reactive to light
- No external signs of head trauma
- Flaccid paralysis of the lower limbs
- Absent patellar reflexes, intact upper limb reflexes
- Sensory level at T4
- Soft abdomen
- No obvious long bone or pelvic injuries
- Normal temperature and blood glucose

Ask the candidate to summarise the case and answer the following questions

- What would you like to do now?
- What imaging is required?
- What is the pathophysiology of neurogenic shock?

## Actor's Instructions:

You are a 25-year-old man who was knocked off your bike and landed on your back. You can remember the incident clearly but now can't move your legs. You are very worried. You also feel a little short of breath and light headed. You have some pain between your shoulder blades but nowhere else.

You are in perfect health and not taking in medications regularly. You do not smoke or take an recreational drugs and drink socially only. You are personal trainer and exercise daily whilst currently training for an ultra marathon. You are terrified you may never be able to work or compete again.

**CRITICAL CARE OSCE - Spinal cord injury**

| Task: | Achieved | Not Achieved |
|---|---|---|
| Introduces self & establishes rapport | | |
| Briefly clarifies history | | |
| Feels hands and pulse | | |
| Asks for pulse rate and blood pressure | | |
| Checks conscious level | | |
| Asks about pain | | |
| Checks pupils | | |
| Assesses limb tone | | |
| Assesses sensation of limbs and torso - identifies sensory level at T4 | | |
| Assesses limb motor function | | |
| Assesses limb reflexes | | |
| Examines abdomen | | |
| Visually inspects long bones/pelvis | | |
| Asks for temperature/glucose | | |
| Responds to patient's concerns appropriately | | |
| Gives patient honest explanation without colluding | | |
| Summarises case to examiner | | |
| States would log roll and assess back/neck/sphincter tone | | |
| Suggests CT or MRI for further investigation | | |
| Can outline pathophysiology of spinal cord injury | | |
| | | |
| Examiner's Global Mark | /5 | |
| Actor / Helper's Global Mark | /5 | |
| Total Station Mark | /30 | |

## Learning Points

- An injury to the spinal cord above T6 may lead to interruption of the sympathetic chain and gives the characteristic cardiovascular picture of bradycardia and hypotension known as neurogenic shock. Paralysis of the intercostal muscles leads to a diaphragmatic breathing pattern. It is important not to mix this diagnosis up with the term 'spinal shock'.

- After completion of the primary survey, urgent imaging is required to identify the lesion and, if appropriate, direct surgical intervention.

- Decreased organ perfusion may lead to organ failure so early recognition and treatment is essential. Judicious fluids, atropine and vasopressor therapy may all be indicated.

# COMMUNICATION SKILLS OSCE –

# Post Herpetic Neuralgia

## Candidate's Instructions:

You are a Foundation Year doctor and are spending the afternoon in the Pain Clinic.
Frances is a 68-year-old woman who has been referred to the clinic by her GP for unremitting pain after an episode of shingles a few months ago.

After 6 minutes the examiner will stop you and ask you to summarise back your findings, suggest your management plan and answer some direct questions.

## Examiner's Instructions:

Frances Smith is a 68-year-old woman who has been referred to the pain clinic by her GP. She has a persistent pain in her lower right chest wall, which has been present since an episode which sounds consistent with Shingles 6 months ago.

The candidate should take a pain history and identify that the likely cause is Post-Herpetic Neuralgia.

If they ask to perform an examination of the patient, acknowledge that this would be relevant, but unnecessary for completion of this station.

With 2 minutes remaining ask the candidate to summarise the case, the potential differential diagnoses and the further management from here.

## Actor's Instructions:

You are a 68-year-old woman who has been referred to the Pain Clinic by your GP. You have been troubled by a pain in the right side of your lower chest for over 6 months now.

It starts in the right side of your back, and shoot round to the ribs in the front of your chest wall, in a narrow band. It began over 6 months ago. It started as an itch, but became painful in a matter of days. You hadn't suffered any injuries to that area.

The pain is always there as an ache or burning, but several times a day it flares up and causes electric shooting pains. Sometimes this happens at night and wakes you up. It doesn't spread or radiate anywhere else. You have not suffered from shortness of breath or a cough. You have not lost any weight, and you don't have any leg swelling.

If asked about a rash, you recall that a few days after the pain started you developed a rash in that area. It was unsightly, blisters which scabbed over after a few days, and very itchy. The rash disappeared after 2 weeks. You put this down to a reaction to some Deep Heat ointment you had applied when the pain initially started. The pain isn't brought on by exercise, nor by eating. If you take a very deep breath the severe electric shooting pain starts.

Your GP has prescribed co-codamol 30/500 2 tablets four times a day. You tend to miss the morning and lunchtime doses if you have plans that day, as they make you groggy. They help a bit, and take the pain from 6/10 to 4/10. At it's worst the pain is 9/10, and then you take 2 tablets of ibuprofen 200mg – you don't think these do much. If asked if you have tried anything else, cold compresses seem to distract you from the pain when it is very bad. You have not tried TENS. You did initially try Deep Heat ointment, but as mentioned above, this seemed to cause a rash so you stopped.

You are a retired teacher. You have given up playing tennis with your friends, as the rubbing of your t-shirt aggravates the pain.

You are otherwise fit and well, on no other medicines, and aren't allergic to anything. You don't smoke, rarely drink, and don't take illicit drugs.

You will be reassured if given a diagnosis which defines this as a neuropathic pain, and told there are specific medications available to treat this type of pain, but dubious if told it is due to a chest infection or injury.

COMMUNICATION SKILLS OSCE – Post Herpetic Neuralgia

| Task: | Achieved | Not Achieved |
|---|---|---|
| Introduces self & establishes rapport | | |
| Briefly clarifies history | | |
| Establishes **s**ite of pain | | |
| Establishes how the pain first began | | |
| Enquires about the **c**haracter of the pain | | |
| Asks about any **r**adiation to other sites | | |
| Asks about **a**ssociated features – shortness of breath, productive cough, leg swelling, rash, weight loss, fever | | |
| Enquires as to **t**iming of pain – any particular time of day | | |
| Asks about **e**xacerbating and relieving factors – eg medications, hot/cold, exercise, relationship to eating | | |
| Establishes **s**everity using a scoring system, e.g. number of out 10 | | |
| Establishes history of rash in dermatomal distribution | | |
| Enquires about impact on mood, working and social life | | |
| Takes a past medical history | | |
| Takes a drug history including allergies | | |
| Takes a social history (smoking/alcohol/illegal drugs) | | |
| Suggests post-herpetic neuralgia as diagnosis | | |
| Discusses management options – anti-neurpathic agents eg pre-gabalin, gabapentin, amitriptyline. TENS, Lidocaine patch | | |
| Suggests sensible differential diagnosis e.g. musculoskeletal pain, pleuritic pain from pneumonia or P.E.,chostocondritis, cholecystitis. | | |
| Addresses patients concerns/answers questions | | |
| Summarises case to examiner | | |
| Examiner's Global Mark | /5 | |
| Actor / Helper's Global Mark | /5 | |
| Total Station Mark | /30 | |

## Learning Points

- Herpes Zoster, or Shingles, causes a vesicular rash, classically in a single unilateral dermatomal distribution. It is caused by re-activation of the Varicella Zoster virus, which is the cause of the common childhood illness "Chicken Pox."

- It can cause neuropathic pain, termed Post Herpetic Neuralgia, particularly in more elderly patients, and can persist for many months. Occasionally Post Herpetic Neuralgia can occur without the preceding rash of Shingles.

- Symptomatic treatment includes use of anti-convulsant medications such as Gabapentin or Pregabalin, or anti-depressant agents such as Amitriptyline. Additionally, the use of TENS or topical agents such as Lidocaine patches may be of benefit.

# COMMUNICATION OSCE – PAIN HISTORY

## Candidate's instructions.

A 38-year-old woman presents to the pain clinic after being referred by her GP for pain in her lower back, gradually worsening over the last year.

You are the Foundation year doctor attached to the clinic and have been asked to take a history from the patient and summarise your findings to the team in view of making a management plan.

After 6 minutes the examiner will stop you and ask you to summarise back your findings, suggest your management plan and answer some direct questions.

## Examiner's instructions

A 38-year-old woman attends the pain clinic complaining of chronic lower back pain.

The Foundation year doctor in the clinic has been asked to take a history from the patient and present to the team. The patient has a history of depression and becomes teary during the consultation.

With 2 minutes remaining ask the candidate to summarise the case, the potential differential diagnoses and the further management from here.

## Actor's instructions

You have been referred to the pain clinic by your GP after multiple visits for lower back over the last year. It is a dull ache that does not move anywhere, there is no history of trauma or injury but you think the pain is getting worse with occasional relief from painkillers.

You have a history of anxiety and depression and have used antidepressants in the past but stopped because you thought they had no effects. You self harmed as a teenager but not in recent years and have no suicidal ideation.

You have changed jobs a few times in the last year because you were not coping under pressure and have recently started a new one where you feel victimised. The low mood has returned with frequents bouts of tears and hopelessness and you are also worried about being overweight. You smoke 15 cigarettes a day and are struggling to quit. You also drink a bottle of wine every night and have done so for the last few months. You do not take any medication, have no allergies and do not use recreational drugs.

You do not have any other physical symptoms, no history of weight loss and problems passing urine or opening bowels. You live alone with no family close by though you speak to them occasionally.

You become teary during the consultation, as you feel frustrated. You also do not think the pain would get better with any intervention and request a sick note to go off work.

**COMMUNICATION OSCE – PAIN HISTORY**

| Task | Achieved | Not Achieved |
|---|---|---|
| Introduces self and gains consent | | |
| Confirms patient's name and date of birth | | |
| Asks about pain using open questions | | |
| Asks about 'red flags' of lower back pain such as weakness, bowel and bladder dysfunction, saddle anaesthesia, weight loss | | |
| Enquires about pain management methods used | | |
| Relevant systems review | | |
| Asks about past medical history | | |
| Asks about drug history and allergies | | |
| Discusses patient's social history including smoking and alcohol | | |
| Explores patient's ideas, concerns and expectations about pain | | |
| Enquires about patient's social support system | | |
| States inappropriateness of giving sick note without attempting to manage pain | | |
| Identifies patient's anxiety and depression as 'yellow flags' | | |
| Offers support for smoking and alcohol misuse | | |
| Asks if patient has questions and ensures ideas and concerns have been explored | | |
| Explains will review case with Pain Consultant and examine patient | | |
| Summarises case with salient points | | |
| Develops appropriate management plan using Bio-Psycho-Social approach | | |
| Empathetic towards patient | | |
| Summarises findings to examiner | | |
| Examiner's global mark | /5 | |
| Actor's global mark | /5 | |
| Total station mark | /30 | |

## Learning Points

- Taking a good history often requires a Bio-Psycho-Social approach to properly understand and appropriately manage patients, as symptoms may not be due to a purely physical cause. This approach can be time consuming in real life clinical scenarios however it is worth investing this time to get a true feel for the issues. Delving into these areas can cause patients to become upset but exploring and identifying these issues will ultimately be in everyone's best interest.

- Knowing the 'red flags' of back pain is essential as may indicate a medical emergency if present. A history of malignancy (no matter how long ago), weight loss, longstanding steroid use, thoracic pain, non mechanical pain, fevers and rigors and urinary retention are some of the key flags to look for.

- Be aware of 'yellow flags', which highlight a patient's risk of developing chronic pain. They include inappropriate attitudes and beliefs about pain, emotional difficulties, problems at work and compensation disputes.

# COMMUNICATION OSCE - Analgesia for labour

## Candidate's Instructions:

You are a Foundation Year doctor on your Anaesthetics rotation. You are spending the day in the labour ward and have been asked to talk to a pregnant woman about the options available for pain relief during labour.

She is a 25 year old primigravida who is 36 weeks pregnant. She has been well during her pregnancy and has no past medical history of note. She is planning to have a normal delivery in the hospital birthing suite.

After 6 minutes the examiner will stop you and ask you to summarise back your findings, suggest your management plan and answer some direct questions.

## Examiner's Instructions:

Lisa is a 25 year old primigravida who has attended the hospital for a midwifery appointment and has asked to speak to a doctor about pain relief during labour.

She is very anxious about the pain of childbirth, but has heard some very worrying stories from friends about the risks of having an epidural. She doesn't know what to do and is getting increasingly worried about having her baby.

The candidate is a Foundation Year doctor who will be expected to explore the patient's concerns and offer simple advice about the options for pain relief during labour in a reassuring and understandable way.

With 2 minutes remaining ask the candidate to summarise the discussion and suggest a plan for this woman.

## Actor's Instructions:

You are Lisa, a 25 year old woman who is 36 weeks pregnant with your first child. As you near your due date, you are becoming increasingly anxious about childbirth, particularly about how you will manage with the pain.

You have several girlfriends who have had epidurals during labour and a few of them went on to have caesarian sections. This has worried you as you've also heard that epidurals can prolong labour. Last week you read a terrible story online about a woman who sustained nerve damage following an epidural and she couldn't walk for 6 months. All these things have really put you off the idea of having one, but you are also terrified of being in pain.

Your partner's mother used to be a midwife and she has told you that in her day women just got on with it and didn't make such a fuss. You're finding that your partner isn't being particularly supportive either, which is making you feel worse.

At your routine midwifery appointment, you decide to ask to speak to a doctor about the options available to you for pain relief during your labour. In addition to exploring the options, you would like to know whether epidurals make you more likely to need a caesarian or prolong your labour.

**COMMUNICATION OSCE – Analgesia for labour**

| Task: | Achieved | Not Achieved |
|---|---|---|
| Introduces self and establishes rapport | | |
| Starts with open questions and allows the patient to talk | | |
| Listens actively and shows empathy | | |
| Clarifies patient's specific concerns about childbirth | | |
| Explores patient's understanding of pain relief available for labour | | |
| Elicits patient's particular concerns about epidurals | | |
| Explains that there are several options available for pain relief – tailored to each patient's needs | | |
| Mentions simple analgesia (paracetamol) | | |
| Mentions gas and air/entonox | | |
| Mentions other pain relief like TENS and water birthing | | |
| Addresses patient's specific concerns about epidural analgesia | | |
| States that epidurals are a very safe technique but acknowledges possible risks | | |
| States that epidural analgesia is the most effective pain relief for labour | | |
| States that epidurals do not increase the risk of caesarian section | | |
| Explains that serious complications of epidurals are very rare | | |
| Offers information leaflet about pain relief during labour | | |
| Offers to refer to a senior anaesthetist if she would like further discussion | | |
| Answers patient's questions in simple language | | |
| Asks about birthing partner and family support | | |
| Summarises findings and options to the examiner | | |
| | | |
| | | |
| Examiner's Global Mark | /5 | |
| Actor / Helper's Global Mark | /5 | |
| Total Station Mark | /30 | |

## Learning Points

- There are numerous ways to provide analgesia for labour, ranging from breathing exercises, massage and family support, to epidurals. No single method is right for every woman and all labour experiences are unique. As healthcare professionals, our job is to provide accurate information that allows our patient's to make informed decisions.

- There remains controversy about epidurals for labour and misinformation about the potential risks is often found online or through child birthing groups. It is a difficult subject in which to design clinical trials and so data is limited, however, what data are available suggest that there is no increased risk of caesarian section after epidurals, though the rate of instrumental delivery may be slightly higher.

- The Obstetric Anaesthetist's association (OAA) provide excellent information leaflets for pregnant women and healthcare professionals which are freely available online (www.labourpains.com).

# COMMUNICATION OSCE – Explaining Anaesthetic drugs

## Candidate's instructions:

You are a Foundation Year doctor on your Anaesthetics rotation. Today there is a year 4 medical student attending your list who has just started the first week of their Anaesthetics rotation. They are interested to talk to you about the different drugs used in Anaesthesia.

Using the labelled syringes/drugs list as an aide memoire, talk the student through the different drugs, giving as much information about each as you can, then answer any questions they may have.

## Examiner's Instructions:

The candidate has been asked to talk to a year 4 medical student about the drugs that are commonly used in Anaesthetics. To help them they should be provided with labelled syringes to use as an aide memoire (or alternatively a list of drugs can be used). The candidate has been instructed to give as much information as they can - the most salient facts are included in the mark scheme.

They will be expected to identify each class of drug and give a brief summary of their clinical usage. They should also field any questions the student may pose

The list of drugs is as follows:

Hypnotics/induction agents
- Propofol
- Thiopental

Opiates
- Fentanyl
- Morphine

Muscle Relaxants
- Suxamethonium
- Rocuronium

Anti-emetics
- Ondansatron
- Cyclizine

Sympathomemetics
- Ephedrine
- Metaraminol

Vagolytics
- Atropine
- Glycopyrollate

Local Anaesthetics
- Lidocaine
- Laevobupivicaine

## Actor's instructions:

You are a 4th year medical student in the first week of your Anaesthetics rotation. Today you are placed on a list with a Foundation Year doctor who you hope will be able to talk you through the drugs that are commonly used in anaesthetics - there seem to be hundreds and you're finding it all a bit confusing!

Ask the candidate if they could tell you what each of the drugs is used for. When they have gone through the drugs ask what is meant by the term 'balanced anaesthesia'. You have a misconception that the drugs used to put the patient to sleep at the start need to last for the whole operation. Ask the candidate 'how do you make sure you give them enough to keep them asleep all the way through? What if the operation takes longer than expected?

**COMMUNICATION OSCE - explaining Anaesthetics drugs**

| Task: | Achieved | Not Achieved |
|---|---|---|
| Introduces self & establishes rapport | | |
| Identifies learning needs of student | | |
| Correctly identifies propofol & thiopental as 'hypnotics'/'induction agents' | | |
| Correctly identifies morphine & fentanyl as 'opiates' | | |
| Explains that morphine is longer acting than fentanyl | | |
| Explains that fentanyl is more potent/stronger than morphine | | |
| Identifies suxamethonium & rocuronium as muscle relaxants | | |
| Explains briefly the difference between depolarizing and non-depolarizing agents | | |
| Identifies ondansatron & cyclizine as antiemetics | | |
| Identifies metaraminol & ephedrine as sympathomemmetics (accept 'drugs that increase the blood pressure) | | |
| Explains that metaraminal & ephedrine act on alpha and beta receptors to have their effect | | |
| Identifies atropine & glycopyrollate as vagolytics/drugs to increase heart rate | | |
| Explains that these drugs block the action of the vagus nerve | | |
| Identifies lidocaine & laevobupivicaine as local anaesthetics | | |
| Explains that these drugs block nerve transmission by blocking sodium channels | | |
| Specifies that local anaesthetics are given by subcutaneous injection or deposited around nerves | | |
| Gives correct definition of 'balanced anaesthesia' (including anaesthesia/analgesia/muscle relaxation) | | |
| Corrects misconception - explains use of volatile/intravenous agents to maintain anaesthesia | | |
| Information pitched and paced appropriately | | |
| Answers students questions clearly | | |
| Examiner's Global Mark | /5 | |
| Actor/Helper's Global Mark | /5 | |
| Total Station Mark | /30 | |

## Learning points:

- A working knowledge of the drugs used in Anaesthesia is useful for all clinicians, especially if you are called upon to assist with the Anaesthetic care of a critically ill patient on the ward or in the Emergency Department - the Anaesthetist is bound to be very grateful for the extra help and it is important for you to known and understand what drugs your patient is having and the ongoing effects they will have on them.

- Induction of general anaesthesia usually involves administration of an intravenous induction agent in combination with a short acting opiate like fentanyl. This combination produces rapid loss of consciousness and obtunds the laryngeal reflexes sufficiently to allow instrumentation of the airway. Muscle relaxants are typically added in order to facilitate endotracheal intubation.

- Before conducting any anaesthetic the Anaesthetist will always prepare their emergency drugs, which must always be readily to hand in order to manage life threatening complications like hypotension, bradycardia or airway obstruction.

# COMMUNICATION – Teaching midwife about spinal anaesthetic

## Candidate's Instructions:

You are a Foundation Year doctor on your anaesthetics placement. On the labour ward a new midwifery student asks you to explain spinal anaesthesia to her.

With 2 minutes remaining the examiner will stop you and ask you some direct questions in regards to spinal anaesthesia.

## Examiner's Instructions:

The candidate has been instructed to explain spinal anaesthesia to a midwifery student.

They should to be able to approach this task by using language and terminology that a junior member of the labour ward team would be expected to understand. The actor has been instructed to seek clarification on a number of points, and may not immediately grasp some concepts. The mark scheme reflects the necessity for a patient approach!

One aspect of this station is to consider the safe conduct of anaesthesia. With 2 minutes remaining ask the candidate directly regarding checks prior to commencing a spinal anaesthetic, patient monitoring during regional anaesthesia, and the emergency management of potential complications after spinal anaesthesia (hypotension and high spinal block). Specific management is not crucial, rather the application of a systematic ABC approach and calling for senior help.

## Actor's Instructions:

You are a first year midwifery student attending the labour ward as part of your clinical experience. This is your second week, and you have been present at a number of normal deliveries but are now going to observe an elective Caesarean section in theatres for the first time. The patient hasn't arrived in the theatre yet, and you want to take the opportunity to ask the anaesthetist about the planned anaesthetic.

You initially have some confusion as you thought all operations are carried out under general anaesthetic and can't believe that the proposed anaesthetic is an awake regional technique. After realising that this is a standard technique you are very inquisitive about the process. You would like to know about the reasons women might select this type of anaesthetic rather than a general anaesthetic, as you would much rather be asleep for any operation. You would also like to know what checks should be carried out prior to performing a spinal.

You know that epidurals are sited in the back and require a lot of clarification as to why a spinal is different to an epidural. Aim to have elements of the process repeatedly explained by the doctor, and ask if you can help by preparing the (incorrect) epidural equipment, such as adhesive tape and epidural drug-delivery pump.

If the doctor becomes impatient, or fails to explain things adequately to your level of understanding this only adds to your level of confusion, and you may become flustered and upset.

**COMMUNICATION – Teaching midwife about spinal anaesthetic**

| Task: | Achieved | Not Achieved |
|---|---|---|
| Introduces self & establishes rapport | | |
| Clarifies identity of midwifery student | | |
| Explains rationale for spinal anaesthetic | | |
| Describes process of siting spinal anaesthetic (positioning, identify level) | | |
| Outlines common drugs used in spinal anaesthetic (local anaesthetic and opiate/strong pain killer) | | |
| Outlines potential problems of GA for LSCS (fetal benefits, aspiration risk) | | |
| Outlines benefits of spinal anaesthetic for elective LSCS (awake patient, partner presence, DVT) | | |
| Explains some differences between spinal and epidural block (needle choice, catheter) | | |
| Acknowledges importance of patient choice and consent for anaesthetic technique | | |
| Indicates requirement for IV cannula | | |
| Indicates requirement for monitoring (ECG, BP, SpO2) | | |
| Indicates requirement for sterility of procedure | | |
| Indicates requirement for presence of a trained assistant | | |
| Indicates requirement for checking blood results (platelets, clotting) prior to commencing | | |
| Indicates requirement to check patient allergy status prior to commencing | | |
| States would ask for senior help in an emergency | | |
| Uses clear language and terminology appropriate for seniority of student | | |
| Clarifies understanding at intervals and doesn't get frustrated at questions from student | | |
| Summarises back to examiner | | |
| Answers questions from examiner in an orderly manner | | |
| | | |
| Examiner's Global Mark | /5 | |
| Actor / Helper's Global Mark | /5 | |
| Total Station Mark | /30 | |

## Learning Points

- Spinal anesthesia is a standard technique in obstetric anaesthesia, and is commonly used for a range of procedures on labour ward. It reduces the risk of DVT and blood loss compared to general anaesthetic, and when used for Caesarean section allows the mother to be conscious and partner to be present at the moment of delivery.

- As doctors we frequently encounter different members of the multidisciplinary team, covering a range of specialties and seniority. Remember that communication skills between professionals are just as important as those with patients. Miscommunication is a common source of error.

- Using the format of "chunks and checks" can be a helpful tool to ensure effective communication when teaching colleagues or describing procedures to patients. Split up the information into sections and confirm understanding before moving on. Remember you don't have to teach everything in one go and setting realistic and achievable learning objectives for the session will lead to a more enjoyable experience for both teacher and learner.

# COMMUNICATION OSCE – EXPLAINING CONSCIOUS SEDATION

## Candidate's instructions:

A 62-year-old man has been admitted under the Gastroenterology team. He is to undergo an elective OGD to investigate his worsening epigastric pain. He vaguely understands the procedure after reading about it on the Internet.

As the Foundation year doctor on the team, you have been asked by a nurse to speak to the patient who has some questions regarding the procedure. He seems to be most worried about being fully awake during it, and would like you to explain how he would be sedated to avoid this.

After 6 minutes the examiner will stop you and ask you to summarise back your findings, suggest your management plan and answer some direct questions.

## Examiner's instructions:

A 62-year-old man is to undergo an elective OGD to investigate his worsening epigastric pain.

The Foundation year doctor has been asked to explain the process of conscious sedation to the patient who is worried about being awake during the procedure. The patient has some prior knowledge about the process as his friend has previously undergone one with a bad experience.

The candidate is to focus on sedation and not necessarily the indication for the OGD.

With 2 minutes remaining ask the candidate to summarise the case, the management so far, and next steps, including the as instructions to be given to the patient after the procedure.

## Actor's instructions:

You are to undergo an OGD after a referral from your GP who is concerned about your history of worsening abdominal pain. The procedure has been explained briefly by your doctor, and you are aware of the indication for it.

You have also discussed it with your friend, who recently had a bad experience during an OGD, as he was awake during the procedure and did not tolerate it well. You are now worried that you will have a similar experience.

A nurse has kindly asked one of the doctors to speak to you about the procedure. You are a non-smoker with no allergies, and drink alcohol socially. You have also been taking antacids over the counter as they relieve your pain. You recently started working as a taxi driver and concerned about being off work. This information is to be provided only when asked directly.

**COMMUNICATION OSCE – EXPLAINING CONSCIOUS SEDATION**

| Task | Achieved | Not Achieved |
|---|---|---|
| Introduces self | | |
| Confirms patient's name and date of birth | | |
| Asks about prior knowledge | | |
| Identifies and addresses patient's concerns | | |
| Explains conscious sedation – informing patient that he will not be intentionally put to sleep but may be drowsy and responsive | | |
| Explains indication for conscious sedation – relaxant and analgesic effect | | |
| Informs patient about fasting | | |
| Asks about medical history, drugs and allergies | | |
| States medication may be given intravenously or intramuscularly | | |
| Explains drugs used are quick-acting and last for short time after procedure | | |
| Discusses risks of conscious sedation – allergic reaction, respiratory depression, hypotension | | |
| Explains patient will be monitored whilst sedated and during recovery | | |
| Briefly discusses process of OGD | | |
| Explains patient should be able to go home soon afterwards | | |
| States patient may return to normal activities the next day | | |
| Ensures patient understands explanation | | |
| Informs patient not to drive or engage in high risk activities for at least 24 hours | | |
| Uses clear sentences, avoiding medical jargon | | |
| Summarises discussion to the examiner | | |
| Answers examiner's question | | |
| Examiner's global mark | /5 | |
| Actor's global mark | /5 | |
| Total station mark | /30 | |

## Learning Points

- It is essential to have good knowledge of common procedures in medicine as well as how to explain them simply but thoroughly to patients. Practicing speaking without the use of medical jargon can go a long way in effectively communicating with patients. In particular be careful with the use of abbreviations that seem second nature to you but may cause confusion to the patient.

- Post procedure instructions should not be neglected as they are often relevant, particularly so in this case where the patient must be advised against driving till the next day. Verbal instructions can often be forgotten so giving written instruction advice is often a recommended adjunct to your discussions.

- Identifying the ideas, concerns and expectations of patients is important in directing the consultation, as information needed may not be what is assumed.

# COMMUNICATION OSCE – Breaking bad news I

## Candidate's instructions:

An 89 year old woman Madelaine has been admitted to the intensive care unit from Emergency Department with a low GCS (6/15) following a massive left sided intracerebral bleed. CT images have been reviewed by the neurosurgical team, who feel that given the extent of the bleed and her current neurological status she is an unsuitable candidate for any neurosurgical intervention. Therefore she will not survive this event.

Her son has arrived at the unit and would like to speak to a doctor before seeing her.

As the senior members are with another patient for the foreseeable future, you as the the foundation doctor in the intensive care team know the patient and details better than anyone else and so have been asked to explain the diagnosis to the patient's son and answer any questions he may have.

## Examiner's Instructions:

An 89 year old woman Madelaine has been admitted to ICU with low GCS (6/15) following a catastrophic left sided intracerebral bleed. She has been discussed with the neurosurgical team and has been deemed not for any neurosurgical intervention and the event is terminal.

Her son has just arrived on the unit aware of the diagnosis and is yet to see the patient. As the senior members are with another patient for the foreseeable future, the foundation doctor in the intensive care team has been asked to explain the diagnosis to the patient's son and answer any questions he may have.

## Actor's Instructions:

You have just arrived on the intensive care unit where your 89 mother Madelaine has been admitted from Emergency Department. You would like to talk to a doctor before seeing her to get an update of her current status.

You were spending the afternoon with your mother when she began complaining of a headache and lost consciousness within a few minutes. You called the ambulance and have come to the hospital alone.

Your mother lives alone and you visit her on alternate weekends. She has hypertension, diabetes and arthritis and regularly forgets to take her medication. She mobilizes with a stick around the house and her neighbor helps her with shopping and cleaning.

In your opinion she was 'well' until today and you have no idea what could have caused her sudden deterioration but gather it is severe as she is in intensive care. You are very anxious to know what the diagnosis is.

Your father in law had a stroke last year and was discharged from hospital 3 months later following rehab. If the doctor does not make it clear that she will not survive this event you ask if she will make a similar recovery.

You take the news badly and you want to be sure that nothing can be done. You ask if nothing is being done due to her age.

**COMMUNICATION OSCE - Breaking bad news I**

| Task: | Achieved | Not Achieved |
|---|---|---|
| Introduces self | | |
| Clarifies who they are speaking to and relationship to patient | | |
| Suggests quite private room and hands bleep to colleague | | |
| Asks nurse to accompany | | |
| Elicits son's current understanding of what has happened | | |
| Elicits son's current ideas, concerns and expectations | | |
| Establish what son would like to know | | |
| Asks if son would like anyone else present | | |
| Gives warning shot | | |
| Gives bad news and allows time before speaking further | | |
| Avoids medical jargon | | |
| Makes it clear that patient will not survive | | |
| Allows for silence | | |
| Allows son to express his emotions | | |
| Demonstrates understanding of Son's confusion in this case compared to family member's stroke and recovery | | |
| Answers Son's questions regarding if this is due to her age | | |
| Summarises conversation | | |
| Asks about religion and offers spiritual support e.g chaplain | | |
| Empathetic throughout but doesn't offer false hope | | |
| Closes consultation appropriately | | |
| Examiner's Global Mark | /5 | |
| Actor / Helper's Global Mark | /5 | |
| Total Station Mark | /30 | |

## Learning Points:

- There is no easy way to deliver bad news and it is important that it is given in a way that patients understand and feel supported. This will vary from patient and family but clarity of message is essential. Taking support in the form of another doctor or nurse is always useful as much for your own wellbeing as the patient and families.

- The challenge in breaking bad news is responding to the range of feelings the individual may be feeling. Silence is a powerful tool in this situation, be sure to wait for cues before moving to the next step of the consultation.

- Using a structured framework such as the SPIKES protocol can be a useful strategy in addressing patients distress and help increase your confidence in delivering bad news

# COMMUNICATION OSCE - Breaking bad news II

## Candidate's Instructions:

Colin Wike, a previously healthy 35-year-old male, was brought to the Emergency Department 4 days ago after suffering a ruptured cerebral aneurysm. Unfortunately he has failed to regain consciousness, remains apnoeic and is currently intubated and ventilated in Intensive Care. His CT brain shows signs of herniation and today on the consultant ward round a plan was made to conduct brainstem testing to confirm the suspected diagnosis of brainstem death.

You are a Foundation Year doctor in the Intensive Care Unit. The patient's wife is waiting to talk to a doctor about her husband's condition and what will happen next.

## Examiner's Instructions:

Colin, a previously healthy 35-year-old male, was brought to the Emergency Department 4 days ago after suffering a ruptured cerebral aneurysm. He has since been cared for on ICU and is currently intubated and ventilated, having shown no signs of recovery. His CT scan shows signs of herniation. The ICU team plan to conduct brainstem testing on him later today.

The patient's wife is waiting to talk to the candidate about her husband's condition. After previous conversations with the team, she is aware that he is gravely unwell and that he is now unlikely to recover.

The candidate's task is to explain the meaning and significance of brainstem death testing in a simple, compassionate and understandable way. The station does not demand that the candidate talk about organ donation.

## Actor's Instructions:

You are the wife of a 35-year-old male who was admitted to hospital following a bleed on the brain whilst at work. You have been happily married for 10 years and have no children. He was taken to the hospital and placed in the Intensive Care Unit (ICU) but has not regained consciousness. You are extremely worried as your husband has been in the ICU for 4 days and has shown no sign of waking. You had a conversation yesterday with one of the ICU doctors and were told that Colin's condition is so serious that he was unlikely to recover.

You are devastated and although your friends and family have been supportive you are despondent as each day you come there is still no improvement in his condition. You are realising that Colin may never wake up and it's hard for you to process all the information, as you still feel in a state of shock. If there is no chance of recovery you know Colin would not want to be kept alive artificially.

The doctor today will inform you that there has been no improvement in Colin's condition and that he is showing signs of profound brain damage. They will tell you that the team will be conducting tests today to see whether any of the vital functions of the brain remain intact. They will tell you that the results of these tests may confirm their suspicion that Colin may be brainstem dead.

You will need clarification on what the diagnosis of brainstem death means and will find it very hard to understand that Colin may have died, but that his heart could still be beating. You should ask the Doctor direct questions about this if they do not address this confusion themselves. The doctor will need to talk through the concepts slowly and compassionately. If you feel overwhelmed with information, you will become very upset and find it impossible to listen to any more.

**COMMUNICATION OSCE - Breaking bad news II**

| | | |
|---|---|---|
| Introduces self and establishes rapport | | |
| Suggests a quiet room and hands bleep to colleague | | |
| Asks for a nurse to accompany | | |
| Asks if patient's wife would like a friend or relative to also be present | | |
| Clarifies relationship to patient | | |
| Elicits wife's current understanding | | |
| Explains that there has been no improvement in Colin's condition | | |
| Explains again how serious Colin's condition is/gives a 'warning shot' | | |
| Explains plan to conduct brainstem testing | | |
| Explains what brainstem death means | | |
| Explains briefly what brainstem death testing entails | | |
| Explains that testing may confirm that Colin is braistem dead | | |
| Clarifies that this means he has died, although his heart may still be beating | | |
| Reassures wife that Colin will be kept comfortable | | |
| Gives information slowly and leaves time for silence | | |
| Avoids medical jargon | | |
| Sensitive and empathic approach | | |
| Checks for understanding | | |
| Answers questions honestly and clearly | | |
| Asks if wife would like to see Colin now | | |
| | | |
| | | |
| Examiner's Global Mark | /5 | |
| Actor / Helper's Global Mark | /5 | |
| Total Station Mark | /30 | |

## Learning Points

- Brain stem death can occur after a variety of pathologies, and its diagnosis requires formal brainstem testing by two doctors, both registered for >5 years, one of whom must be a consultant.

- The distinction between 'Brainstem Death' and 'Circulatory Death' is complex and must be explained clearly to patient's relatives.

- When dealing with grieving families it is important not to overwhelm them with complex information. Their raw emotional state can make it very difficult to process and recall what they are told. In this example, the conversation about brainstem death would already be overwhelming for the patient's wife - don't be tempted to include organ donation in this conversation as well! In clinical practice it is often necessary to have several difficult conversations with relatives, breaking bad news in stages and allowing everything to sink in.

# COMMUNICATION SKILLS OSCE - Patient with chronic pain

## Candidate's Instructions:

Richard is a 56-year-old man who has presented to the pre-assessment clinic in preparation for an elective umbilical hernia repair under general anaesthetic.

You are a Foundation Year1 doctor on your anaesthetics rotation and have been asked to come and talk to Richard by one of the pre-assessment nurses. He suffers with a chronic pain condition and he would like to talk about pain management around the time of his operation.

Please take a pain history and answer any questions that the patient may have.

After 6 minutes the examiner will stop you and ask you to summarise back your findings and suggest your management plan.

## Examiner's Instructions:

Richard is a 56-year-old man who has presented for elective umbilical hernia repair under general anaesthetic.

He has a long standing history of complex regional pain syndrome following a motorcycle accident and injury to his left arm 7 years ago. His pain prevents him from working and he takes several analgesics.

After six minutes stop the the candidate and ask them to summarise the case and the important issues. Ask them about features of chronic pain and the principles in managing chronic pain perioperatively.

## Actor's Instructions:

You are a 56-year-old man who has presented for elective umbilical hernia repair under general anaesthetic.

You have a long standing history of chronic pain following a motorcycle accident and injury to your left arm 7 years ago. Your pain prevents you from working and you take many analgesics including paracetamol, ibuprofen, amitriptyline, lidocaine patches and oramorph prn. The main symptoms you experience are burning, shooting, tingling pain in your left arm, which sometimes feels alternately cool and hot. You sometimes find that even putting on a shirt in the morning hurts your arm. The arm becomes swollen sometimes and you have noticed changes in the pattern of hair growth. You occasionally smoke cannabis to help with the pain. You drink a few pints of beer each day.

Although you are very keen to have your operation, you are concerned about your pain control afterwards, and in particular what will happen if you miss your medication doses.

**COMMUNICATION OSCE - Patient with chronic pain**

| Task: | Achieved | Not Achieved |
|---|---|---|
| Introduces self & establishes rapport | | |
| Clarifies planned procedure | | |
| Asks about site of pain | | |
| Asks about onset of pain | | |
| Establishes ongoing, chronic pain | | |
| Establishes neuropathic nature (character of pain - burning/shooting/electric shock) | | |
| Asks about associated features e.g. skin changes | | |
| Asks about injury to the arm | | |
| Asks about exacerbating factors | | |
| Asks about relieving factors | | |
| Takes a drug history including allergies | | |
| Asks about impact upon work, finance | | |
| Asks about mental health | | |
| Asks about social functioning | | |
| Asks about drugs and alcohol | | |
| Addresses patient concerns and expectations | | |
| Explains medications can be continued throughout the perioperative period | | |
| Comes to a sensible plan about post-operative analgesia, mentions local anaesthesia | | |
| Summarises case to examiner | | |
| Is able to identify features of chronic pain | | |
| | | |
| Examiner's Global Mark | /5 | |
| Actor / Helper's Global Mark | /5 | |
| Total Station Mark | /30 | |

## Learning Points

- Chronic pain is often defined as pain persisting for longer than three months. It often has a 'neuropathic' element which is described as burning, shooting or tingling in nature.

- Its long term nature can unfortunately lead to profound upset to the patient's functional ability, and there may be elements of depression, financial uncertainty and difficulty forming and maintaining relationships.

- Peri-operative pain management can be challenging, and the analgesic plan should address the chronic pain (which often means continuing the patient's current medications), as well as the acute pain relating to surgery. Multimodal approaches and advice from the pain team are invaluable.

# COMMUNICATION SKILLS OSCE – Awareness Under Anaesthetic

## Candidate's Instructions:

You are the Foundation Year doctor on the Surgical Admissions Unit. You have been asked to clerk in Emily, a healthy 42 year old who is listed for a laparoscopic cholecystectomy later today. The nursing staff have warned you that she seems very nervous about having a general anaesthetic. Please take a relevant history and explore the patient's concerns and expectations.

After 6 minutes the examiner will stop you and ask you to summarise back your findings, suggest your management plan and answer some direct questions.

## Examiner's Instructions:

Emily, is a healthy 42-year-old who is listed for a laparoscopic cholecystectomy later today. The nursing staff are aware that she is very nervous about having a general anaesthetic, as she believes she suffered from an episode of "awareness" during a previous anaesthetic.

The candidate should undertake a standard medical and anaesthetic history, but should focus specifically on Emily's concerns about awareness. Where possible they should offer reassurance, and make a plan to have her reviewed by an anaesthetist.

In the final 2 minutes, ask them to summarise the case. If they have not mentioned it already, ask if they are aware of the quoted incidence of awareness in the NAP 5 study, and if they know of any specific devices which monitor depth of anaesthesia.

## Actor's Instructions:

You are a healthy 42-year-old woman who is listed for a laparoscopic cholecystectomy later today
When you were 28, you sadly suffered from a ruptured ectopic pregnancy, and had to undergo an emergency salpingectomy (removal of a Fallopian tube.)
You had a general anaesthetic, but are sure you remember part of the procedure you shouldn't. You recall the sensation of being moved from one bed to another, and hearing voices discussing starting a blood transfusion because of your low blood pressure. You felt very panicked as you feared the operation was about to start, but you couldn't move to tell anyone you were awake. You remember nothing further until waking in recovery.
You were so traumatized by the loss of the pregnancy, that you didn't discuss the episode of awareness with anyone at the time. For several months afterwards you suffered from flashbacks and nightmares, which have recurred while you have been awaiting this operation.
You are worried that you are "resistant" to anaesthetics, and that it could be even worse this time. You have read in the newspapers about people being awake during surgery and feeling the pain of the procedure.
If you don't feel you are believed, or perceive that the candidate is unsympathetic towards your concerns, you will become upset and state that you won't have your operation.
You will feel reassured if it is explained to you that there were risk factors for awareness during your last anaesthetic – (emergency case, significant blood loss), which are absent on this occasion.
You will also feel reassured if you hear about the careful monitoring and presence of an anaesthetist throughout the case, particularly if the candidate states they will arrange for the anaesthetist to come and speak to you.

**ANAESTHETIC COMMUNICATION SKILLS OSCE – Awareness Under Anaesthetic**

| Task: | Achieved | Not Achieved |
|---|---|---|
| Introduces self & establishes rapport | | |
| Clarifies planned procedure and indication | | |
| Asks about previous anaesthetics | | |
| Takes a medical history – cardiovascular/respiratory/systemic enquiry | | |
| Takes a drug history including allergies | | |
| Takes a social history (smoking/alcohol/illegal drugs) | | |
| Takes a family history (including problems with general anaesthesia) | | |
| Asks about fasting status | | |
| Identifies episode of possible awareness from patient's history | | |
| Asks questions to establish extent of awareness and whether patient experienced awareness with pain | | |
| Asks about psychological, social and emotional impact of the episode of awareness | | |
| Demonstrates empathy | | |
| Discusses risk factors for awareness – emergency case, cardiovascular instability, use of muscle relaxant | | |
| Provides reassurance about monitoring for signs of awareness – ECG and NIBP, End Tidal Gas Monitoring, clinical signs, presence of anaesthetist | | |
| Addresses patients concerns/answers questions | | |
| Shows some knowledge of depth of anaesthesia monitoring e.g. BIS | | |
| Makes plan to refer patient to anaesthetist for further discussion | | |
| Suggests follow up with GP or counselling service | | |
| Summarises case to examiner | | |
| Shows some awareness of the NAP 5 study and quoted incident of awareness being 1:19 000 | | |
| | | |
| Examiner's Global Mark | /5 | |
| Actor / Helper's Global Mark | /5 | |
| Total Station Mark | /30 | |

## Learning Point:

- The National Audit Project 5 (NAP 5) estimates that the incidence of Accidental Awareness during General Anaesthesia occurs in 1:19 000 general anaesthetics.

- Over 40% of patients who experience awareness go on to develop significant psychological morbidity. Clearly this cohort will need ongoing attention to ensure they have been supported in dealing with this.

- Depth of Anaesthesia monitors have been developed which use adaptations of EEG monitoring or Auditory Evoked Potentials have been developed, but their routine use has not yet been recommended by the Royal College of Anaesthetists.

# CLINICAL SKILLS OSCE - Pre operative check and application of monitoring

## Candidate's Instructions:

Nigel is a 70-year-old man who has presented for left knee replacement under spinal anaesthesia. He has just arrived in the anaesthetic room.

You are a Foundation Year1 doctor on your anaesthetics rotation and you have been asked to ensure that the correct patient has arrived for the correct operation. You should then apply the pulse oximeter, ECG and perform non-invasive blood pressure (NIBP) measurement.

After 6 minutes the examiner will stop you and ask you to summarise back your findings and ask you some direct questions.

## Examiner's Instructions:

Nigel is a 70-year-old man who has presented for knee replacement under spinal anaesthesia.

The candidate should verify the patient's identity and consent, including the side of surgery. They should then apply and obtain baseline observations including pulse oximetry, ECG and non-invasive blood pressure (NIBP).

- The pulse is 70/min and regular
- The ECG appears normal
- NIBP is 140/80

Ask the candidate to summarise their findings and ask the following questions;

- Please comment on the patient's observations
- Can you name two other questions are asked at 'sign in'?
- What are the other parts of the WHO surgical checklist called and when are they performed?

## Actor's Instructions:

You are a 70-year-old man presenting for surgery to replace your left knee. You are fit and well and have been waiting for this operation for over 12 months so are very keen to get on with it today. You know friends that have had the same operation and it all seemed to have gone very smoothly so you have no concerns.

If asked:

- You can confirm you signed the consent form this morning
- You have no allergies
- You last ate and drank over 6 hours ago
- You have no questions

**CLINICAL SKILLS OSCE: Pre operative check and application of monitoring**

| Task: | Achieved | Not Achieved |
|---|---|---|
| Introduces self & establishes rapport | | |
| Cleans hands and wears gloves | | |
| Checks the patient's name | | |
| Identifies two name bands | | |
| Checks the patient's date of birth | | |
| Checks the patient's ID number against the consent form | | |
| Verifies the patient understands the operation she is having | | |
| Confirms the correct operation on the consent form | | |
| Verifies the date of the consent form | | |
| Verifies the patient's signature on the consent form | | |
| Checks that there is an indelible mark on the left leg | | |
| Applies the pulse oximeter | | |
| Correctly applies the ECG leads whilst preserving dignity | | |
| Chooses an appropriately sized blood pressure cuff | | |
| Measures non invasive blood pressure | | |
| Shows awareness of potential for discomfort during blood pressure reading | | |
| Summarises case to examiner | | |
| Identifies normal observations | | |
| Is aware of other questions on WHO checklist - any two from: 2*group and save, fasting status, airway risks, anaesthetic machine check, drug chart reviewed, allergy status | | |
| Can name the other parts of the process – time out (before skin incision) and sign out (before the patient leaves the operating room) | | |
| Examiner's Global Mark | /5 | |
| Actor / Helper's Global Mark | /5 | |
| Total Station Mark | /30 | |

## Learning Points

- In the UK in 2009, there were approximately 150,000 reports of patient safety issues relating to surgery. Wrong patient and wrong site surgery is classed as a 'never event' by the NHS.

- The WHO '5 steps to safer surgery' consists of a pre-operative briefing, sign in, time out, sign out and debrief.

- By following the 5 steps, it is thought that health care professionals can reduce the occurrence of the most common and avoidable risks to patients undergoing surgery.

# CLINICAL SKILLS OSCES: Oxygen delivery devices

## Candidate's Instructions:

You are the Foundation Year1 on your anaesthetics placement. You have a third year medical student with you on a clinical attachment. Your consultant has asked you to provide some brief teaching to the student regarding the provision of oxygen to patients.

Review the following diagrams of oxygen delivery devices. These can be used as a reference point for your teaching.

After 6 minutes the examiner will stop you and ask you questions regarding the delivery of oxygen.

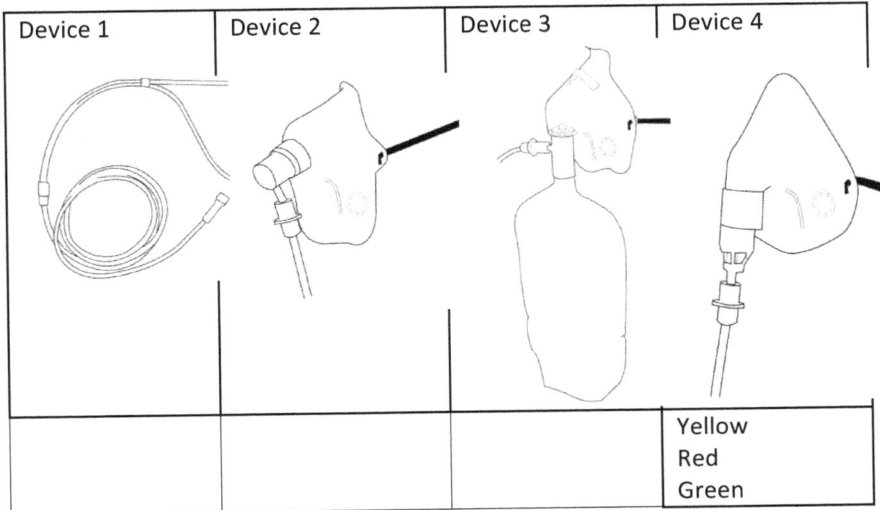

## Examiner's Instructions:

The candidate should review the diagrams of 4 oxygen delivery devices. They should then provide brief teaching to the medical student, including some of the advantages and disadvantages of each oxygen delivery device. Some points in the accompanying mark scheme will be covered during the teaching.

With 2 minutes remaining in the station directly ask the candidate any of the following questions that have not already been explained /answered. These form two parts; the first part relates to the achievable oxygen concentrations offered by each device, the second part consists of 4 clinical scenarios.

The answers regarding oxygen concentrations are provided as absolute figures. In reality there is a wide degree of variation in oxygen concentrations, so these values (apart from atmospheric oxygen) can be considered as estimates. Answers within 2% are acceptable.

The text in italics after each clinical scenario is for information purposes and can be reviewed with the candidate after the station has been completed if time allows.

Questions:
1) As a percentage, what is the atmospheric concentration of oxygen (i.e., that found in room air)?
21%.

2) Identify Device 1: Nasal cannulae / speculae

3) What percentage of oxygen will the patient receive if this device is attached to oxygen at 2 L/min?
~28%

4) And at 6 L/min?
~38%
5) Identify Device 2: Hudson mask / face mask

6) What percentage of oxygen will the patient receive if this device is attached to oxygen at 6 L/min?
~50%

7) Identify Device 3: Reservoir mask / non-rebreathe mask

8) What percentage of oxygen will the patient receive if this device is attached to oxygen at 15 L/min?
90%

9) How do you inflate the reservoir bag after the mask is attached to an oxygen supply before applying the mask to the patient?
Occlude the valve inside the mask.

10) Identify Device 4: Venturi mask

11) These devices have colour-coded adapters to control the inspired concentration of oxygen. For each of the colours listed in the table can you indicate the oxygen percentage each should supply?
Yellow 35% Red 40% Green 60%

12) What else relating to oxygen supply allows the device to administer the specified oxygen percentage?
Oxygen flow rate.

13) Where can the appropriate flow rate for each adapter be found?
It is printed on the collar of the Venturi attachment.

14) Which of the above devices are 'fixed performance devices'?
Venturi mask only.

## Clinical scenarios

For each of the following scenarios choose the most appropriate device.

Scenario 1: 24-hours post-operatively, a patient on the surgical ward has an $SpO_2$ of 93%. They are comfortable and have a normal respiratory rate.
Answer: Nasal cannulae.

*The incidence of atelectasis post operatively leads to a short-term additional FiO2 requirement. In this instance the most practical choice best tolerated by the patient would be nasal cannulae.*

Scenario 2: A patient with severe COPD has presented with an exacerbation of his disease. He is responding to nebulised treatment, and requires an arterial blood gas sample.
Answer: Venturi face mask.

*Controlled oxygen therapy is important for patients with severe COPD. As the disease progresses, there may be chronic hypercapnoea which can affect the sensitivity of the brainstem's respiratory centres to changes in PaCO2. A small proportion of these patients may rely on relative hypoxia to maintain their respiratory effort - the 'hypoxic drive'. Venturi masks play an important role in providing supplemental oxygen in these situations especially.*

Scenario 3: A patient admitted into the Emergency Department resuscitation area as a trauma call after a road traffic collision, with chest wall bruising and an obvious femoral fracture.
Answer: Reservoir / non-rebreathe mask.

*This patient may have significant chest wall and pulmonary injuries, with blood loss from the femoral injury. Until the injury pattern is fully elucidated the patient should receive maximal oxygen therapy.*

Scenario 4: A normally fit and well patient recovering in the endoscopy department after a colonoscopy under light sedation. Answer: Hudson face mask.

*Procedural sedation can result in a temporarily reduced respiratory drive. The most practical device to administer supplemental oxygen in the short term for a drowsy patient is the face mask.*

## Actor's Instructions:

You are a third-year medical student on an anaesthetics attachment. It is your first day in the anaesthetic room and would like some teaching on the basics of oxygen delivery. You have been on medical and surgical placements in hospital, so have seen different types of masks used to give patients oxygen, but don't feel confident as to which device should be used when. You would like to ask the Foundation Year1 doctor the names of each of the devices, and some clarification as to their usage.

In particular, enquire about the what the tubing should be attached to (you have seen different gas supplies on the wall, and cylinders used as well). For each device you'd like to know some of their advantages and disadvantages. Review the examiner's instructions at this point, as some content will be covered during direct questioning from the examiner.

**CLINICAL SKILLS OSCE: Oxygen delivery devices**

| Task: | Achieved | Not Achieved |
|---|---|---|
| Introduces self and establishes learning environment | | |
| 1) Can define atmospheric $O_2$ concentration (21%) | | |
| 2) Correctly identifies nasal cannulae | | |
| 3) States delivers ~ 28% $O_2$ at 2 L/min | | |
| 4) States delivers ~ 38% $O_2$ at 6 L/min | | |
| 5) Correctly identifies Hudson mask | | |
| 6) States delivers ~50% $O_2$ at 6 L/min | | |
| 7) Correctly identifies reservoir / non-rebreathe mask | | |
| 8) States delivers ~ 90% $O_2$ at 15 L/min | | |
| 9) States valve held down to inflate reservoir before applying to the patient | | |
| 10) Correctly identifies Venturi mask | | |
| 11) States $FiO_2$ delivery of Venturi attachments | | |
| 12) States specific oxygen flow rate determines $FiO_2$ | | |
| 13) States Venturi flow rate can be found on collar of adapter (also accept: packaging) | | |
| 14) Fixed performance device: Venturi mask only | | |
| Elaborates advantages / disadvantages for devices | | |
| Scenario 1: Nasal cannulae selected | | |
| Scenario 2: Venturi mask selected | | |
| Scenario 3: Reservoir mask selected | | |
| Scenario 4: Hudson face mask selected | | |
| | | |
| Examiner's Global Mark | /5 | |
| Actor / Helper's Mark | /5 | |
| Total Station Mark | /30 | |

## Learning Points

- The amount of oxygen a patient receives using any device is dependent on a range of patient factors. Variables such as the pattern of breathing, respiratory rate, route (nasal or mouth breathing) and device tolerance can lead to wide variations in actual inspired oxygen concentrations.

- As with any device or piece of medical equipment, it is important to be aware of the correct usage of oxygen delivery devices and the need to prescribe oxygen. It is also useful to be aware of their limitations. Oxygen is too important to get wrong!

- The normal peak inspiratory flow rate for an adult is around 30 L/min. Most oxygen supplies (wall and cylinder) have a maximum flow rate of 15 L/min. To allow concentrations of close to 100% to be delivered to the patient, the reservoir mask supplements the shortfall from the supply. For this reason, the reservoir must be inflated before it is applied to the patient.

# CLINICAL SKILLS OSCE: Setting up IV infusion

## Candidate's Instructions:

You are the Foundation Year doctor on call. You have been called to see Lindsey, a 19 year old girl who has been fitting on the ward for 10 minutes despite a total of 8mg lorazepam. You recognise she is in status epilepticus and call the anaesthetic registrar on call. The anaesthetic registrar advises you to immediately start a phenytoin infusion whilst they make their way to the ward.

Using the BNF calculate the dose of phenytoin and set up the IV infusion

Lindsey  Hosp No: N66234
DOB: 21/09/1997
Weight 65kg
NKDA

## Examiner's Instructions:

The candidate is the Foundation Year1 on call . They have been called to see Lindsey, a19 year old girl who is in status epilepticus. They have been advised by the anesthetic registrar to immediately start a phenytoin infusion.

Using the BNF the candidate will calculate the dose of phenytoin and set up the IV infusion

Lindsey  Hosp No: N66234
DOB: 21/09/1997
Weight 65kg
NKDA

**CLINICAL SKILLS OSCE: Setting up an IV infusion**

| Task: | Achieved | Not Achieved |
|---|---|---|
| Confirms correct patient's chart and checks allergy status | | |
| Prescribes phenytoin at dose of 18-20mg/kg | | |
| Prescribes phenytoin as infusion in 0.9% sodium chloride | | |
| Prescribes at rate 10ml/min | | |
| Rate does not exceed 50mg/min | | |
| Prescription signed | | |
| Prescription legible | | |
| Decontaminates hands and wears gloves | | |
| Concentration phenytoin 50mg/ml (5 ml ampoule) | | |
| Checks expiry date of phenytoin | | |
| Draws up phenytoinin 50ml luer lock syringe | | |
| Checks expiry date of 0.9% sodium chloride | | |
| Dilutes phenytoin in 45ml 0.9% sodium chloride | | |
| Primes extension with 0.9% sodium chloride and checks for air bubbles | | |
| Attaches extension to syringe | | |
| Loads 50ml syringe into pump | | |
| Checks cannula is safe to be used | | |
| Cleans cannula with alcohol wipe prior to attaching extension | | |
| Ensures pump device is set correctly according to the prescription | | |
| Starts Pump | | |
| | | |
| Examiner's Global Mark | /5 | |
| Actor / Helper's Global Mark | /5 | |
| Total Station Mark | /30 | |

## Learning Points

- Infusion rate (ml/hr)= dose rate (mg/h) / Concentration (mg/ml)

- It's a common misconception that the preparation and administration of drugs is a 'nursing job'. This is certainly not the case in Anaesthetics, but every doctor should be able to perform these tasks competently. Being confident in using equipment like syringe pumps, and preparing medication can be especially important in emergency situations like this one.

- For most syringe pumps the rate is set in ml per hour however for some syringe drivers the rate is set according to the distance travelled by the plunger in mm per hour or mm per 24 hour- Always be sure to check units before setting the rate to avoid fatal errors.

# CLINICAL SKILLS OSCE – Management of acute post operative pain

## Candidate's Instructions:

You are the foundation year doctor in anaesthetics and you have been called to recovery to review Betty.

Betty is an 80 year old female who had a left total hip replacement under general anaesthetic 2 hour ago and is now reporting pain. According to the Anaesthetic record, she received 8mg of morphine IV intra-operatively, but no other analgesia.

In addition, the recovery nurse points out that the patient's drug chart has not been completed.

Please review the patient's pain and prescribe appropriate treatment.

## Examiner's Instructions:

The candidate is the foundation year doctor in anaesthetic and has been called to recovery to review Betty an 80 year old lady who is 2 hours post left total hip replacement.

She is currently reporting pain in her left hip and has been given no medication since leaving theatre. She received 8mg IV morphine on the table, but no other analgesia.

The candidate is expected to review her pain and prescribe appropriate treatment.

## Actor's Instructions:

You are Betty, an 80 year old lady who has undergone a left total hip replacement under general anaesthetic. You came around from the anaesthetic 2 hours ago and felt ok initially, but have developed increasingly severe pain over the last half an hour.

You are currently experiencing 5/10 pain in your hip at rest and 6/10 pain when you try move your leg.

PMH:
Osteoarthritis, Hypertension, Hypercholestrolaemia, Peptic ulcer

DH:
Allergic to penicillin- rash
Co-codamol 30/500 1-2 tablets QDS
Amlodipine 5mg
Simvastatin 40mg OD
Omeprazole 20mg OD

**CLINICAL SKILLS OSCE - Management of acute post operative pain**

| Task: | Achieved | Not Achieved |
|---|---|---|
| Introduces self | | |
| Confirms patient is in pain | | |
| Assesses severity of pain | | |
| Asks for/says they would check patient's observations (HR/BP/SpO2) | | |
| Checks past medical history | | |
| Checks drug history | | |
| Confirms allergies | | |
| Documents allergies on chart | | |
| Prescribes regular paracetamol 1g QDS | | |
| Does not prescribe an NSAID | | |
| Prescribes appropriate regular weak opiate | | |
| Appropriate regular dose and interval of weak opiate | | |
| Prescribes PRN strong opiate for breakthrough pain | | |
| Appropriate PRN dose and interval for strong opiate | | |
| Prescribes PRN antiemetic | | |
| Prescribes 2 different classes of antiemetic | | |
| Prescribes Naloxone | | |
| Prescribes PRN laxative | | |
| Writes legibly | | |
| Prescription signed and dated | | |
| | | |
| | | |
| Examiner's Global Mark | /5 | |
| Actor / Helper's Global Mark | /5 | |
| Total Station Mark | /30 | |

## Learning Points

- The WHO analgesic ladder is an excellent framework for managing acute pain and is core knowledge for any new Doctor starting on the wards - go and learn it if you haven't already!

- 'Multi-modal analgesia' is the term we use to describe an analgesic strategy that combines multiple drugs of different classes. In combination these drugs are more effective than they would be in isolation - in this regard they are said to act 'synergistically'.

- Non steroidal anti-inflammatory drugs (NSAIDs) can be extremely effective additions to your multimodal analgesic strategy. However, they are not benign substances and some of the side-effects are potentially serious. Renal impairment is a particular concern in the elderly, or in those patients with other risk factors for acute kidney injury (AKI) in whom NSAIDs are to be avoided.

# CLINICAL SKILLS OSCE - Opioid Conversion

## Candidate's Instructions:

Clarice is a 60-year-old woman who was admitted for mastectomy for breast cancer. Her postoperative pain has been managed with IV morphine PCA, with a bolus dose of 1mg. She has used a total of 20mg in the last 24 hours. Her postoperative biochemistry is normal.

You are a Foundation Year doctor on your anaesthetics rotation and you have been asked to prescribe an appropriate dose of modified release morphine tablets, with some additional opioid for breakthrough pain. You may ask the patient questions you feel are relevant.

After 6 minutes the examiner will stop you and ask you to summarise back your drug chart and ask you to answer some direct questions.

A summary of Clarice's drug chart is shown below:

| MANOR PARK NHS FOUNDATION TRUST<br><br>WARD DRUG CHART | Mrs. Clarice<br><br>6579-091A<br><br>3-4-1956 | Allergy status: | | | |
|---|---|---|---|---|---|
| | | | 23/9/16 | 24/9/16 | 25/9/16 |
| *REGUALAR MEDICATIONS* | Paracetamol 1g qds | 6 | * | | |
| | | 12 | * | | |
| | | 18 | * | | |
| | | 22 | * | | |
| *PRN MEDICATIONS* | Morphine PCA<br>1mg bolus<br>5 minute lockout<br>No background infusion | 6 | * | | |
| | | 12 | * | | |
| | | 18 | * | | |
| | | 22 | * | | |

## Examiner's Instructions:

Clarice is a 60-year-old woman who was admitted for mastectomy for breast cancer. Her postoperative pain has been managed with IV morphine patient controlled analgesia system (PCA), with a bolus dose of 1mg. She has used a total of 20mg in the last 24 hours.

The candidate should take a pain history (including allergies) and formulate a pain management plan that should include a prescription for an appropriate dose of oral morphine.

Ask the candidate the following questions:

- What other medications may be useful to administer in this scenario?
- What emergency drug should also be prescribed?
- What advice would you give the patient?

## Actor's Instructions:

You are a 60-year-old woman who was admitted for mastectomy for breast cancer. Your post operative pain has been managed quite well using IV morphine PCA and you are keen to transition to oral medication so you can be freed up from the some of the wires! You feel some discomfort around the wound and nowhere else. If you had to score your pain out of ten you would say '2' at rest and '5' when you cough or try to get up.

You have a little nausea and feel a bit 'bunged up'; you haven't opened your bowels in 3 days. You have taken ibuprofen before with no problems and have been eating and drinking well so far.

You have no allergies and have not taken oral morphine before.

You have no other co-morbidities.

**CLINICAL SKILLS OSCE - Opioid Conversion**

| Task: | Achieved | Not Achieved |
|---|---|---|
| Introduces self & establishes rapport | | |
| Verifies identity of the patient and that the drug chart is for the correct patient | | |
| Takes a focused pain history | | |
| Attempts to assess pain severity | | |
| Elicits history of constipation | | |
| Elicits history of mild nausea | | |
| Asks about allergies | | |
| Asks about other co-morbidities | | |
| Asks about oral intake | | |
| Asks about history of taking oral analgesics | | |
| States would complete allergy section of drug chart | | |
| Prescribes appropriate dose of modified release morphine tablets (accept 20mg – 30mg bd of MST) | | |
| Prescribes appropriate dose of immediate release morphine for breakthrough pain (e.g. oramorph or sevredol 10-20mg 2-4 hourly). | | |
| Explains analgesic plan to the patient | | |
| Suggests the addition of laxatives | | |
| Suggests the addition of antiemetics | | |
| Highlights the potential for other analgesics to be used e.g. short term ibuprofen | | |
| Suggests the addition of naloxone as an emergency drug | | |
| Explains the importance of good analgesia and that regular review will be undertaken | | |
| Summarises case to examiner and answers questions | | |
| | | |
| Examiner's Global Mark | /5 | |
| Actor / Helper's Global Mark | /5 | |
| Total Station Mark | /30 | |

## Learning Points

- Effective postoperative analgesia is crucial in postoperative mobilization and recovery. The responsibility for this lies not only with the anaesthetists but with the doctors looking after the patient post operatively on the ward.

- Intravenous morphine can be converted to oral morphine at a ratio of 1:2-3, so that 10mg of IV morphine is equivalent to 20-30mg of oral morphine. As well as a 'maintenance' dose, a breakthrough prescription should also be completed (for adults, 10-20mg of immediate release morphine is a good starting point).

- Opioids can have troublesome side effects including constipation and nausea that may themselves hinder recovery, so it's often a good idea to make sure that concurrent antimetics and laxatives are also prescribed and that the patient is warned to look out for these adverse side effects.

# CLINICAL SKILLS OSCE – IV CANNULATION

## Candidate's instructions.

A 17-year-old girl presents to the ED with persistent vomiting and diarrhoea causing significant dehydration. She appears very anxious about being in hospital.

You are the Foundation year doctor in the medical team and have been asked to insert a cannula in the patient to administer intravenous fluids.

## Examiner's instructions

A 17-year-old girl presents to the ED with persistent vomiting and diarrhoea (secondary to gastroenteritis) causing significant dehydration. She appears very anxious about being in hospital.

The Foundation year doctor has been asked to insert a cannula in order to administer intravenous fluids. The patient will become distressed, as she is frightened of needles and will attempt to refuse the procedure. The candidate is to identify this and adequately explain the procedure and the indication for it, addressing any concerns she may have.

Afterwards the candidate is to insert a cannula into the simulation mannequin using an aseptic and safe technique. Check for proper disposal of equipment.

## Actor's instructions

You have presented to the ED after 2 days of persistent vomiting and diarrhoea that came on after eating a takeaway. This is your first time attending hospital and you are anxious about what will happen. You are also frightened of needles and will try to avoid them as much as you can. The nurse has told you that the doctor might put a needle in to give you fluids and you are very frightened.

A doctor, who appears to be young, is seeing you making you more worried about their experience performing the procedure. You initially refuse and ask about alternatives. You remain persistent until the procedure is explained and you are reassured about the need for it.

The procedure goes well to your surprise and afterwards you ask how long the cannula would remain in for.

**CLINICAL SKILLS OSCE – IV CANNULATION**

| Task | Achieved | Not Achieved |
|---|---|---|
| Introduces self | | |
| Confirms patient's name and date of birth | | |
| Explains procedure and gains consent | | |
| Identifies and addresses patient's concerns regarding pain allowing time for questions | | |
| Gathers and prepares all equipment required – alcohol swab, tourniquet, cannula, sharps bin, gauze, 0.9% saline, syringe, cannula dressing | | |
| Washes hands | | |
| Exposes patient and identifies site | | |
| Puts on gloves | | |
| Applies tourniquet and palpates vein | | |
| Cleans skin with alcohol swab and does not repalpate site | | |
| Pulls skin taut in preparation for cannula | | |
| Informs patient before inserting needle | | |
| Looks for flashback then advances cannula while withdrawing needle | | |
| Disposes of needle in sharps bin and caps cannula | | |
| Flushes cannula with 0.9% saline | | |
| Applies dressing with date | | |
| Disposes of used equipment in clinical waste bin | | |
| Removes gloves and washes hands | | |
| Appropriately answers cannula would remain for maximum of 72 hours | | |
| Remains calm and professional during patient interaction | | |
| | | |
| Examiner's global mark | /5 | |
| Actor's global mark | /5 | |
| Total station mark | /30 | |

## Learning Points

- Intravenous cannulation is an essential procedure as a junior doctor. Regular practice as a student will go a long way to developing and building confidence in this skill. Nobody is infallible though so if you are unsuccessful on a patient on numerous occasions then don't be too proud to ask for help.

- Establishing rapport with patients using good communication skills can be effective in identifying and addressing their concerns, thereby improving patients' experiences.

- Remember that in order to perform procedures properly, a safe environment is important before and afterwards. Aseptic techniques and proper disposal of equipment should not be disregarded.

# CLINICAL SKILLS OSCE – FLUID PRESCRIPTION

## Candidate's instructions:

A 75 year old female, Sophie (D.O.B. 23/12/41, MRN 00123456), has been brought in to the emergency department with a 2 day history of diarrhoea and vomiting.

She has a past medical history of hypertension and diabetes and usually takes the following medications:

Ramipril 5mg OD
Frusemide 20mg OD
Metformin 500mg TDS
Aspirin 75mg OD

She is allergic to penicillin which causes a rash.

You are the Foundation Year Doctor on call covering the medical wards. You have been asked to rewrite the patient's drug chart as the original copy has gone missing. The nurse on the ward has also asked you to prescribe some intravenous fluids as the patient is still not tolerating much oral intake. The nurse can provide you with further information about the patient should you require it.

After 6 minutes the examiner will stop you and ask you to summarise back your work, and ask you to answer some direct questions.

## Examiner's instructions:

The candidate is a Foundation Year doctor covering the medical wards. They have been asked by a staff nurse to rewrite the drug chart of a patient whose original chart has gone missing. The patient also needs a prescription for intravenous fluids as she is not tolerating oral intake.

The patient is a 75 year old female who has been admitted after a 2 day history of severe diarrhoea and vomiting. She has a past medical history of hypertension and diabetes for which she usually takes Ramipril, metformin, frusemide and aspirin. She is allergic to penicillin which causes a rash.

The candidate will be expected to acquire additional information before completing the prescription chart. The staff nurse has printed a copy of the U&Es and has performed a set of physiological observations. This information will be given by the nurse if the candidate asks for it. The candidate should make a brief assessment of the patient (a simulation mannequin) though you should inform them that a full history and examination is not required for completion of this station. The station should be equipped with gloves and apron to emphasise the infection control issues relevant to a case of diarrhoea and vomiting. In addition to hand decontamination with alcohol gel, the candidate should also state that they would wash their hands with soap and water after contact with a patient with D&V.

The candidate should enter the correct identification information and allergy status into the drug chart. They should also indicate on the chart that the patient's antihypertensives and hypoglycaemic agents are to be omitted pending further medical review.

Finally, they should recognise severe hypokalaemia and prescribe appropriate intravenous potassium replacement.

In the final 2 minutes ask the candidate to summarise the case then ask the following questions:

1)What is the maximum rate of potassium replacement via a peripheral cannula?

2)What further action needs to be taken to ensure patient safety in this case?

3)What are the ECG features of severe hypokalaemia?

## Actor's Instructions:

You are a staff nurse on a medical ward looking after Sophie, a 75 year old female who has been admitted with diarrhoea and vomiting.

Shortly after her arrival on the ward, you noticed that the patient's drug chart was missing and contacted the F1 doctor to come and rewrite it.

You have printed off some blood results and have performed an initial set of physiological observations. You should provide the candidate with this information only if they ask for it. If the candidate asks to assess the patient they can demonstrate their assessment on a simulation mannequin to which you should direct them. The patient does not have a urinary catheter and if asked you are able to insert one. There is an IV cannula in situ which was inserted in the Emergency Department. You have checked that it is patent and ready to use.

Observations:

| | |
|---|---|
| HR | 90bpm |
| BP | 110/57 |
| RR | 18 |
| Temp | 36.5 |
| GCS | 15 |
| BM | 7.4mmol/L |

Blood results:

| | |
|---|---|
| Sodium | 136mmol/L |
| Potassium | 2.8mmol/L |
| Creatinine | 95 mol/L |
| Urea | 8.7mmol/L |

**CLINICAL SKILLS OSCE – FLUID PRESCRIPTION**

| Task | Achieved | Not Achieved |
|---|---|---|
| Introduces self | | |
| Wears gloves and apron | | |
| Takes focussed history from patient | | |
| Asks for patient's physiological observations | | |
| Asks for patient's blood results | | |
| Identifies hypokalamiea | | |
| Requests 12 lead ECG | | |
| Requests insertion of urinary catheter and completion of fluid balance chart | | |
| Establishes presence of patent IV cannula | | |
| Completes identification correctly on drug chart | | |
| Completes penicillin allergy status including severity - rash | | |
| Prescribes regular medications | | |
| Indicates ramipril, metformin and frusemide are to be held pending medical review | | |
| Prescribes appropriate IV potassium replacement (accept 1-2 litres NaCl each with 20-40mmol KCl over 2-6 hours) | | |
| States would wash hands with soap and water following encounter | | |
| Summaries case to examiner | | |
| Knows maximum rate of peripheral potassium replacement - 20mmol/hr | | |
| Suggests patient needs ongoing potassium replacement with regular measurement of serum potassium | | |
| States will refer for urgent senior review | | |
| Knows ECG features of hypokalaemia (prolonged PR/ST depression/T-wave inversion/U-waves) | | |
| Examiner's global mark | /5 | |
| Actor's global mark | /5 | |
| Total station mark | /30 | |

## Learning Points

- The job of an F1 doctor on call can be extremely busy. You will often be called upon to perform administrative tasks like rewriting drug charts or prescribing IV fluids, sometimes without all the salient clinical information put in front of you. This case demonstrates that prescribing fluids is just as important as prescribing any other drug - failing to recognise and treat severe hypokalaemia can have life-threatening consequences. Remember to always check the patient's U&Es before prescribing IV fluids!

- Severe hypokalaemia (< 3mmol/l) has characteristic ECG changes (increased PR interval, T-wave inversion, ST depression, U-waves). It also predisposes to life-threatening arrhythmias.

- Giving intravenous potassium comes with it's own risks as rapid changes in serum potassium concentration may also cause arrhythmias. In the ward setting, the concentration of potassium in intravenous fluids should not exceed 40mmol/L, and should be given at a rate no faster than 20mmol/hr. If the patient requires more rapid correction, this should occur in a monitored, critical care area via central venous cannula.

# CLINICAL SKILLS OSCE –
# Checking and administering a blood transfusion

## Candidate's Instructions:

You are the Foundation Year1 doctor on your Anaesthetics rotation. Your consultant has asked you to assist in recovery where a patient from your list needs a blood transfusion following their elective colorectal procedure. The patient is haemodynamically stable and has a haemoglobin level of 75g/L.

Your consultant has prescribed 1 unit of packed red cells to be transfused. You are required to check and administer the blood with a member of staff in recovery.

After 6 minutes the examiner will stop you and ask you to summarise back your case, and ask you to answer some direct questions.

## Examiner's Instructions:

The candidate is a Foundation Year doctor on their Anaesthetics rotation. They have been asked to check and administer a blood transfusion to a patient who is in recovery after his elective colorectal procedure this morning.

The candidate must safely check and prepare the unit of blood for administration, assisted by the recovery nurse.

With 2 minutes remaining at the end of the station the candidate may require direct questioning regarding frequency of observations during transfusion and time limits for product administration after removal from temperature controlled storage.

## Actor's Instructions:

You are an experienced recovery nurse who is competent in checking and administering blood products. You should check the patient's identity, prescription, and the blood unit label with the candidate.

You are particularly aware that patients should undergo 3-point confirmation of identity prior to proceeding (Name, DOB, and Unit Number)

You remember on previous occasions using a special blood giving-set. The unit has been appropriately prescribed to run over a duration of 3 hours.

You have just performed observations on the patient. The patient's pulse rate is 78 beats per minute, blood pressure 133/81 mmHg, respiratory rate 19, and temperature 36.3 degrees centigrade. The patient's cannula is patent and working well.

The porters brought the blood unit to recovery (out of the blood bank fridge) 20 minutes ago. You would like to know what to do if the transfusion takes longer than the prescribed three hours as you are aware of guidance to complete transfusion within four hours of the blood product leaving controlled temperature storage.

## *Resources*

*Patient Band with 3-point ID: Name, DOB, Unit Number*

*Mock up of blood component label: with 3-point ID, blood type, date, +/- Unit Number.*

*Relevant section of blood product prescription chart (patient info and section with prescription)*

**CLINICAL SKILLS OSCE – Checking and administering a blood transfusion**

| Task: | Achieved | Not Achieved |
|---|---|---|
| Introduces self | | |
| Clarifies Identity of patient : Name | | |
| Clarifies Identity of patient : Date of Birth | | |
| Clarifies Identity of patient : Patient Number | | |
| Cross-checks 3-point identity with prescription chart | | |
| Cross-checks identity with blood product label | | |
| Checks group of blood unit | | |
| Checks expiry date of blood unit | | |
| Performs two-person checks | | |
| Reviews appropriate duration of administration | | |
| Ensures suitable cannula in situ and functioning | | |
| Ensures appropriate blood giving set available (filter giving set) | | |
| Enquires about consent for receiving blood transfusion | | |
| Checks for any allergies | | |
| Visually inspects unit for damage / precipitants | | |
| Requests / asks to review pre-transfusion observations (pulse rate, blood pressure, respiratory rate, temperature) | | |
| Advises set of observations 15 minutes after start of transfusion | | |
| Advises set of observations 60 minutes post-transfusion | | |
| Aware of maximum time for blood to be out of fridge before return to blood bank when asked | | |
| Summarises case to examiner and answers questions | | |
| Examiner's Global Mark | /5 | |
| Actor / Helper's Global Mark | /5 | |
| Total Station Mark | /30 | |

## Learning Points

- Serious complications of blood transfusion are rare. Most incidents of wrong-product transfusion are related to human error; therefore, most centres employ 2-person checks of the patient identity and blood product prior to administration. Positive patient identification requires "3-point verification". This is usually full name, date of birth, and a unique identifier number.

- Blood banks keep packed red cells in temperature controlled storage until they are ready to be transfused. Once units have left the blood bank they must be kept in an insulated storage box to maintain a safe temperature and have completed transfusion within a 4-hour limit. They can be returned to controlled temperature storage within 30 minutes if no longer required.

- A failsafe way to avoid transfusion complications is to avoid unnecessary transfusions altogether – most hospital blood banks will produce guidelines regarding appropriate use of blood transfusion.

# ANAESTHETIC SKILLS OSCE – Basic Airway Management

## Candidate's Instructions:

Michelle is a 26-year-old woman who has returned to the Gastroenterology ward following a colonoscopy under sedation.

You are a Foundation Year doctor on the ward and you have been called over by the nurse, who is unhappy that Michelle seems very drowsy and is snoring. Her respiratory rate is 6 breaths/minute.

Please use the mannequin to demonstrate the manoeuvers you would perform and equipment you would use to support her airway.

## Examiner's Instructions:

Michelle is a 26-year-old woman who has returned to the GI ward following a colonoscopy under sedation.

The nurse on the ward is unhappy that Michelle seems very drowsy and is snoring. Her respiratory rate is 6 breaths/minute.

Ask the candidate to address the partial airway obstruction by demonstrating on the mannequin some simple airway manoeuvers, correctly sizing and inserting airway adjuncts, and demonstrating they can use the bag-valve mask to support ventilation.

Any requests to know what sedation the patient has received (100mcg of fentanyl, 4mg of midazolam) or obtain antagonists such as naloxone or flumazenil should be acknowledged, but keep them focused on the practical aspects of the station.

They should ask for help, and should be assured that whatever assistance they request is on its way, but they need to continue to manage the patient until that help arrives.

## Assistant's Instructions:

You are the nurse on the GI ward, and are concerned that this patient who has just returned from a colonoscopy is drowsy and making snoring sounds.

You have noticed from the colonoscopy notes that she has received 100mcg of fentanyl and 4 mg of midazolam.

If asked, you report that her respiratory rate is 6 breaths/minute, and her SpO2 on room air is 90%.

The candidate should try to get a response from the patient, the patient will grimace and make some flexion movements with her upper limbs, but won't open her eyes and will continue to snore. (GCS 6 E1V1M4)

If the candidate performs the initial airway manoeuvers correctly and applies 15L of oxygen via a non-rebreathe mask, you may inform them that the SpO2 is now 98%.

To move the candidate through the station, tell them that the patient is still snoring when the nasopharyngeal airway is inserted. They should move on to insert an oropharyngeal airway. If this is inserted correctly, tell them that the snoring has stopped. If they ask, tell them that the chest and abdomen are moving in synchrony, that the mask is misting/they can feel breath on their cheek. However, re-enforce that the respiratory rate is only 6 breaths/minute. If they do not move on to assist the patient's breathing with the self-inflating bag, prompt them by stating the respiratory rate is now 4 breaths/minute and that the SpO2 is 92%.

The final task the candidate should perform is the insertion of an iGel, if they do not move on to perform this themselves you may prompt them – "do you want to insert a Supraglottic Airway Device? That would free our hands from holding the mask."

You may assist the candidate by passing them any pieces of equipment which they ask you for. They may also ask you to squeeze the self-inflating bag, or assist with mouth opening or jaw thrust during insertion of the Supraglottic Airway Device/iGel.

If you are asked to summon help, or obtain specific drugs such as naloxone or flumazenil, assure them that you have made the request and that these things are on their way.

Equipment Requirements:

Mannequin with working airway anatomy and lungs which will expand.
Non-rebreathe O2 mask
Face Mask and Self-Inflating Bag
Nasopharyngeal Airways in Sizes 6, 7 and 8.
Lubricant gel
Oropharyngeal Airways in Sizes 2, 3 and 4
iGel Supraglottic Airway Devices in Sizes 3, 4 and 5

**ANAESTHETIC SKILLS OSCE – Airway Manoeuvres**

| Task: | Achieved | Not Achieved |
|---|---|---|
| Checks safe to approach and tries to rouse patient using shake and shout | | |
| Calls for help – senior doctor/fast bleep anaesthetist/2222 crash call | | |
| Correctly demonstrates head tilt/chin lift (no history of C-spine trauma) | | |
| Correctly demonstrates jaw thrust | | |
| Selects correct size of nasopharyngeal airway for mannequin (Size 6 or 7 most women, Size 7 or 8 most men) | | |
| Correctly inserts nasopharyngeal airway, after applying lubricant | | |
| Demonstrates how to size an oropharyngeal airway – flange level with incisors, tip to angle of jaw | | |
| Selects appropriate size of oropharyngeal airway for mannequin | | |
| Demonstrates correct insertion technique for oropharyngeal airway – careful placement, upside down until encounters resistance from hard palate, rotates 180 degrees | | |
| Requests and applies 15L O2 with non-rebreath mask. Does not use self-inflating bag to provide oxygen while patient spontaneously breathing | | |
| States how would assess for improvement – no more snoring, synchrony of chest and abdominal wall movements, look, listen and feel for effective breathing | | |
| Correctly applies face mask – chin to bridge of nose covered, no pressure on eyes, correct placement of hand(s) to hold mask – C-shape with around mask, lifting mandible forward with free fingers | | |
| Successfully uses self-inflating bag to demonstrate chest rise – can ask assistant to squeeze bag if 2 hands needed to hold mask | | |
| Requests the self-inflating bag be connected to 15L of O2 | | |
| Demonstrates appropriate rate of ventilation – 12-16 breaths/minute | | |

| | | |
|---|---|---|
| Selects appropriate size of iGel SAD, 4 for most patients as suggested by weight range written on device | | |
| Demonstrates correct insertion technique – opens mouth, SAD correct way up, careful insertion into mouth, firm pressure until device comes to natural stop (May ask for jaw thrust from assistant) | | |
| Correctly attaches self-inflating bag to SAD and demonstrates adequate chest rise | | |
| Requests appropriate monitoring – minimum $SpO_2$ probe, others could include ECG, NIBP, End Tidal $CO_2$ | | |
| Suggests further management options – one or more of antagonists (naloxone, flumazenil) definitive airway management by anaesthetist, HDU/ICU admission | | |
| Examiner's Global Mark | /5 | |
| Actor / Helper's Global Mark | /5 | |
| Total Station Mark | /30 | |

## Learning Points

- Airway obstruction and respiratory depression can occur following sedation

- A self-inflating bag contains a one-way valve, which causes high resistance to breathing and makes it unsuitable for spontaneously ventilating patients.

- Supraglottic Airway Devices form a seal above the larynx, reducing gastric distension from ventilation attempts with the self-inflating bag. The second generation devices such as the iGel also allow passage of a gastric tube, allowing the emptying of stomach contents.

CPSIA information can be obtained
at www.ICGtesting.com
Printed in the USA
LVHW080905080219
606760LV00036B/982/P

9 780990 853862